Big Fat Keto Lies

Table of Contents

What the Experts are Saying

*M*arty Kendall enjoys one of the highest vantage points of the entire nutritional landscape.

Thanks to an open mind and a keen eye for spotting data patterns, Marty has managed to entirely reverse-engineer eating.

In his book, 'Big Fat Keto Lies', Marty sifts through the quagmire of diet religion and deftly plucks all of the essential gems out of a huge pile of unhelpful dietary dogma.

In my humble opinion, he is definitely one of the best and brightest minds in the entire nutrition space at the moment. I would recommend his book to anyone, but especially anyone in the low-carb/keto space. Really timely.

Ted Naiman, MD

Marty, this book is brilliant! This is my message to the world also!

You continue to inform people with honest and accurate information and self-experimentation. We are all learning together. Thank you for your contributions.

Nutrient density is where it's at, and I agree entirely that each person needs to figure out their own carbohydrate tolerance.

Professor Mark Cucuzzella MD FAAFP
Professor West Virginia University School of Medicine
WVU Centre for Diabetes and Metabolic Health

Marty's fresh take on the value of data as it pertains to fasting stopped me in my tracks. It is the proverbial missing piece of the puzzle for so many. His contributions to nutrition science and patient care are extraordinary.

Cynthia Thurlow
Nurse Practitioner
Everyday Wellness

There are many myths and misconceptions about low-carb and ketogenic diets. Learning how to do the diet correctly from the beginning will make a big difference, especially on your medium to long-term results and health.

Keto can be a great tool to improve your health, but more so if done correctly from the start. In his book, Marty does an excellent job at reviewing, correcting and explaining, in an easy-to-understand way, the most prevalent myths in the low-carb/keto community.

Luis Villaseñor
Nutritionist, SFN
KetoGains Founder

Big Fat Keto Lies is a must-read for anyone who has stalled on their path to health and optimal weight. Data-driven engineer Marty Kendall unpacks the common keto dietary conventions that typically cause people to fail in the long term.

Marty, through easy-to-follow discussions, explains the often neglected but important practice of focusing on dense foods to control appetite beyond simply looking at macros and calories.

If optimising your health and nutrition is your goal, you will not be disappointed.

Jeffry Gerber, MD
Family Physician, Denver's Diet Doctor
Denver Colorado, USA

Marty is the best. Like a watchmaker who understands every tiny cog and wheel of nutrition.

Cian Foley

Don't Eat for Winter

Every popular diet contains some truth and, as time goes on, ever greater outlandish, hyperbolic and inaccurate claims. Marty Kendall does a superb job at dispelling the many myths of the keto diet that have grown up over the past few years, but offers us a legitimate solution based on his analysis of many large data sets.

Big Fat Keto Lies is an essential read for anyone wanting to step out of all pop-culture diet trends and embrace a truly agnostic form of nutrition for health.

Aimee Gallo

Vibrance Nutrition

Certified Nutritionist

Masters in Nutrition and Functional Medicine

If your goal is to healthfully lose body fat using the most up-to-date nutrition science and don't know where to start, I highly recommend Big Fat Keto Lies by Marty Kendall.

As a Harvard-trained radiation oncologist, integrative oncologist and functional medicine practitioner, I have spent nearly two decades counselling patients on the importance of reducing body fat and insulin resistance. During this time, I have witnessed countless patients try unsuccessfully to lose weight or maintain their weight loss using the latest "fad diets" (including the popular ketogenic diet and intermittent fasting). Once you read Big Fat Keto Lies, you will understand why these approaches often don't work.

Marty explains, in a very approachable manner, the reasons why people are biologically programmed to fail on most weight-loss diets or calorie restriction. In Big Fat Keto Lies, you will also learn practical, effective, healthful and sustainable approaches to fat loss that are simple to understand and implement. I will be recommending this book for all of my patients who want to optimise their metabolic health, lose body fat and improve their anti-cancer biological terrain.

Dr Brian Lawenda, MD
Medical Director, Northwest Cancer Clinic
Director of Integrative Oncology and Cancer Survivorship
GenesisCare, Kennewick, WA

Marty's new book on 'keto lies' demonstrates a very deep understanding of fundamental ideas in nutrition and metabolism. Great stuff Marty!

RD Dikeman, PhD
Type One Grit

Introduction

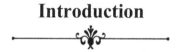

T he last thing the world needs is another keto diet book.
Right?

Wrong!

Welcome to Big Fat Keto Lies!

This book is a tour of the most prevalent keto and low-carb myths and misconceptions, and my learnings gleaned through my quest for nutritional enlightenment in 'Ketoland'.

Like many others, I was once a loyal keto disciple, following the latest keto diet gurus during my early quest for nutritional enlightenment.

I could quote chapter and verse from the latest best-selling keto bible. But what I *couldn't* do, no matter *how* religiously I kept the faith, was lose weight—much less fat—or improve my blood glucose and other critical biomarkers.

What I *don't* want to be with **Big Fat Keto Lies** is another false prophet that people blindly follow. Instead, I hope to take the role of shepherd and tutor, guiding you—just as I did myself, my family, and now thousands of Optimisers in our Optimising Nutrition community—by exposing the **big fat keto lies** that I once believed but have unlearned on my journey.

The story of how 'low-carb' morphed into 'keto' is a classic example of the 'if a little is good, more must be better' mentality that we often fall victim to.

But 'keto-bashing' isn't the purpose of *Big Fat Keto Lies*. There are numerous benefits from a lower-carbohydrate diet that enables to avoid the hyperpalatable, processed, and nutrient-poor combination of fat and carbs that drives us to now eat more than ever!

Sadly, I fear that many of the invaluable aspects of a lower-carb diet will be lost when the trend dies and keto becomes another dietary fad and a 'thing of the past'.

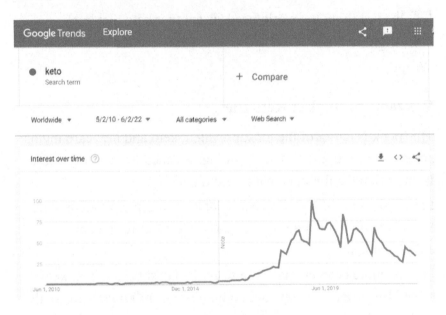

My goal with *Big Fat Keto Lies* is to help you leverage the many benefits of a lower-carb way of eating by exposing, correcting, and clarifying keto beliefs that have proven to be counterproductive and even dangerous when taken to extremes.

The nutritional framework detailed in this book will empower you with awareness to be a fiercely objective consumer, deputised to ferret out half-baked truths and outright lies in any social, electronic, digital, or print media that crosses your path.

While many of you may have already acquired these detective skills, many 'Ketonians' have not (yet!). Sadly, it's often the most devout keto true believers that often end up with the *least* optimal results. The injustice comes down to splinter groups, subcultures, and closed-minded communities postulating their "one true way"."

It is no wonder that confusion is rife, and inflammatory online arguments continue to spark like wildfire. However, these e-wars have ironically boosted the popularity of these keto half-truths because 'controversy gets clicks'.

We now have endless bastardised versions of keto. A leaky revival tent has taken the place of the core benefits of a lower-carb diet.

Objections to Big Fat Keto Lies

Since Big Fat Keto Lies was initially released, several readers have pushed back, claiming that many keto advocates now already agree with the "12 lies".

This is partly true, and some of the keto gurus have quietly backed away from some of the lies. A few brave and noble leaders have publicly renounced their previously held beliefs.

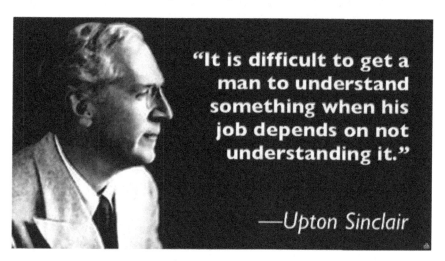

"It is difficult to get a man to understand something when his job depends on not understanding it."

—Upton Sinclair

But confusion will prevail until a united council of keto gurus admits to their faithful disciples that 'these are the truths we once believed but have now been proven false'.

You can either:

- hold your breath, waiting for the hierarchy to release an updated 'official' version of the keto gospel and recant the errors of the past, or
- you can get busy reading to understand how you can optimise your diet to suit *your* unique goals and context.

I've organised the chapters of **Big Fat Keto Lies** around 12 of the most rampant keto 'commandments' that tend to cause the most confusion and failure.

- Keto Lie #1: 'Optimal ketosis' is a goal. More ketones are better.
- Keto Lie #2: You have to be 'in ketosis' to burn fat.
- Keto Lie #3: You should eat more fat to burn more body fat.
- Keto Lie #4: Protein should be avoided due to gluconeogenesis.
- Keto Lie #5: Fat is a 'free food' because it doesn't elicit an insulin response.
- Keto Lie #6: Food quality is not important. It's all about insulin and avoiding carbs.
- Keto Lie #7: Fasting for longer is better.
- Keto Lie #8: 'Insulin toxicity' is enemy No. 1.
- Keto Lie #9: Calories don't count.
- Keto Lie #10: Stable blood sugars will lead to fat loss.
- Keto Lie #11: You should 'eat fat to satiety' to lose body fat.
- Keto Lie #12: If in doubt, keep calm and keto on.

Charitable readers might consider these 'half facts/half fictions' as no more than a dozen innocuous, misguided, and misconstrued 'little white lies.'

But diligently following these 'commandments' often leads one to fail to achieve their health goals of reducing body fat, achieving healthy blood sugar levels, or optimising their metabolic health.

Those gullible enough to 'go keto' based solely on what they have 'learned' through social media, podcasts, or by 'eavesdropping' on the endless arguments on Facebook, Twitter, Instagram, and TikTok put themselves at risk of endangering their own health.

Similar to how the commercial diet industry profits by pedalling its wares to desperate dieters, the charming and persuasive 'snake oil' front men and women hawk their pseudo 'keto' vendibles to consumers desperate to hand over their hard-earned cash for that elusive 'magic pill'.

In an attempt to cut through the noise, I have taken a data-driven approach to identify factors like satiety, nutrient density, and healthy blood glucose levels that make any diet work.

Once you understand these fundamental principles of nutrition, you will be able to identify extremes like chasing higher ketones, more fat, and the extremes of plant vs animals in your diet that are not only irrelevant but counterproductive and often dangerous if taken too far.

When you examine each "lie" through the lens of Nutritional Optimisation, you'll find clarity, a basic understanding of keto mechanics, answers to frequently asked questions, and practical action steps to take when—or if—you discover your keto beliefs no longer serve you.

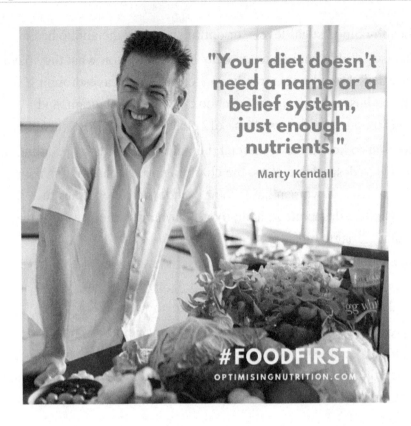

"Your diet doesn't need a name or a belief system, just enough nutrients."

Marty Kendall

#FOODFIRST
OPTIMISINGNUTRITION.COM

Who Am I?

My name is Marty Kendall.

I live in Brisbane, Australia.

I'm not a doctor.

I'm an engineer.

I have a family history of obesity and diabetes. I was always the 'fat kid'.

My family was primarily vegetarian for religious reasons, so I ate plenty of processed grains and fake meat way before it was popular.

I am married to my wife Monica, who happens to have Type-1 Diabetes.

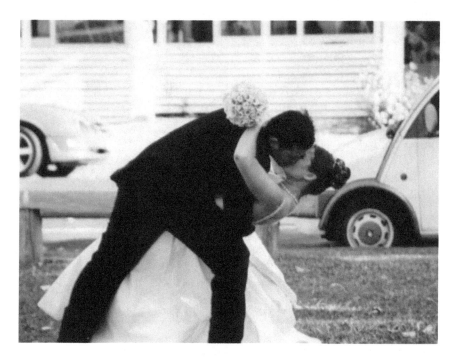

My quest to understand nutrition, diabetes, insulin and optimal blood sugar management began in 2002 when we started dreaming of having kids. We wanted to avoid the scary array of complications that often accompany high blood sugars during pregnancy.

We now happily have two robust, healthy teenagers!

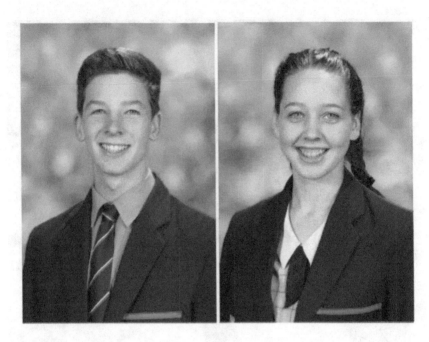

By experimenting with different dietary modifications, we have managed to halve Monica's daily insulin requirements. The adventure has also changed us.

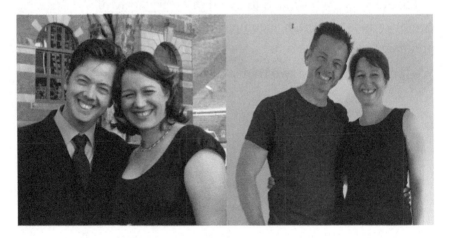

As an engineer, I think in numbers, charts, and systems. What you're reading is not a typical diet book. *Big Fat Keto Lies* lays out the *logic* of how various health and nutrition parameters interact.

Having access to several large and unique datasets allowed me to test various nutrition theories for myself. I wanted to identify the shared themes that make all diets work and eliminate the 'magical thinking' and belief—not to mention the ethical and commercial bias—that is so common in nutrition and other 'soft' fields.

Through my excursions and explorations of nutrition-focused literature, data, analysis, and research, I collected some unique insights that I can't wait to share with you.

I hope these insights will keep you from stumbling headlong into the pitfalls and potholes (and rabbit holes, too) that swallow up too many folks travelling down their road to nutritional enlightenment.

Insights from Type-1 Diabetes

I spend a lot my day watching Moni's continuous glucose meter (CGM) trace as I fine-tune her closed-loop insulin pump system to optimise her blood sugars. I'll admit, I'm obsessively fascinated by this!

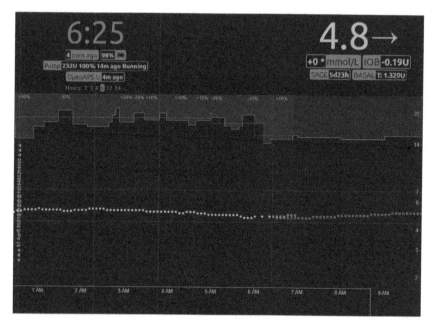

I want to understand how I can empower Monica to optimise control of her diabetes, manage my health, and set an example for our kids.

I have used my analysis skills to crunch the numbers to give Monica the best chance at a long, healthy, and vibrant life. It's super satisfying to see her now living with a non-diabetic HbA1c of 5.1% with around 30 units of insulin per day, compared to an HbA1c greater than 7% and 50-60 units per day that she started with.

I consider this an honour because I have learned so much about the various factors that affect insulin and blood sugar. People with Type-1 Diabetes give us fascinating quantitative insight into how our bodies respond to the food we eat.

I have also learned that it is critical to understand the difference between someone with Type-1 Diabetes and the 98.5% of us with fully functioning pancreases.

Sadly, the majority of the keto doctors have lost sight of this and fail to consider the factors like body fat levels and other variables unrelated to food that influence basal insulin requirements and the critical difference between *exogenous* (injected) insulin and *endogenous* insulin (produced by your body).

The techniques that help people with Type-1 Diabetes stabilise their insulin and blood sugars do not necessarily lead to optimal health and fat loss for the rest of us.

Despite what we believe, most of us can't turn off our pancreas to stop producing insulin regardless of what we eat. Unfortunately, this critical subtlety seems to be lost or ignored by many low-carb and keto-savvy leaders, gurus, and doctors.

What is Agnostic Nutrition?

In days gone by, humans interpreted things they didn't understand as mysterious or magical. We formed religions and cult-worshipped the sun, earth, fire, thunder, and rain as *deities* that gave us nourishment and sustained us.

In modern times, we abandoned many of the old *deities* as we gained more insight into the elements of nature. Empirical data and a deeper scientific understanding have since filled many of our knowledge gaps.

While we have gained a deeper understanding of the external world and universe, many of the things that occur *inside* our bodies are still a mystery to us.

We may no longer attribute natural phenomena to the interventions of the gods, but that hasn't stopped many of us from ascribing near 'magical' or 'supernatural' powers to *diets*.

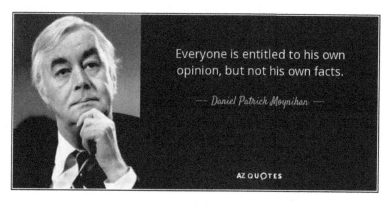

Everyone is entitled to his own opinion, but not his own facts.

— Daniel Patrick Moynihan —

AZ QUOTES

While nutrition is still an *evolving* science, it is still a science with finite principles and *not* a matter of religious belief or debate. While commercial interests and religious perspectives have heavily influenced the conversation around nutrition, I believe nutrition science needs to be agnostic. There must be fundamental principles that apply to all humans.

Context is critical. To make progress towards your destination, you need to understand where you are now and where you want to go. My aim in this book is to highlight the most powerful levers in nutrition and show you how they can be applied to various contexts for different people with different goals.

Endogenous Ketosis for Health and Fat Loss vs Therapeutic Ketosis

Nutrition is not a ' 'one-size-fits-all' solution. To ensure you get the desired outcome on a ketogenic diet, it is critical to understand the difference between:

- a ketogenic diet designed for optimal health, weight loss, and diabetes reversal to achieve endogenous ketosis when fat is released from your body stores to be used for energy, and
- a therapeutic ketogenic diet designed for the management of epilepsy, Parkinson's, dementia, and Alzheimer's disease where ketone levels are derived from dietary fat or exogenous ketone supplements.

Simply 'going keto' by adding more fat or chasing higher ketones may not get you closer to your goal of improved metabolic health. In fact, it could lead you further away from your goal if you don't tailor your nutritional approach to your current context and intentions.

Optimising Nutrition

In January 2015, I started sharing my observations on OptimisingNutrition.com and was overwhelmed by the responses. In addition to writing articles, I spent a lot of time analysing people's food logs to create recommendations that helped them move towards more optimal nutrition.

Three years ago, Alex Zotov contacted me out of the blue. He offered to partner with me to develop a suite of tools that would help automate and scale Nutritional Optimisation to help more people.

Alex is a programmer with a background in neuroscience and app creation for doctors and researchers that are user-friendly. After gaining weight after his professional tennis career, he was also on a quest to solve the puzzle of nutrition quantitatively.

Over the past four years, we have helped people apply the insights from our analysis by developing the Nutrient Optimiser.

Peter Schimke
I have only just joined and working my way through it and this may be one of the most comprehensive, user-focused, gentle (you won't believe how important that is) tools I have ever encountered. It is logically set up. There is clear structure, pathway and purpose. And there is a nod to all areas of the science of nutrition, including the psychological and behavioural. I am really impressed. A tool genuinely designed for the user. Thanks.

1 h   Like   Reply   3

We have run numerous Masterclasses and have seen some radical results in people who have implemented our systemised approach to personalised nutrition by managing the metrics that matter.

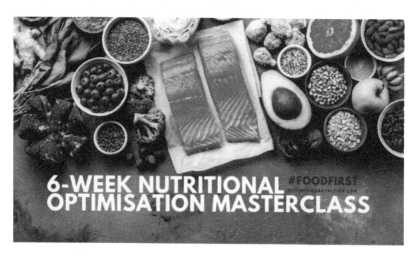

In an effort to bring <u>Nutritional Optimisation</u> to the masses, we have continued to refine our data-driven approach to nutrition to make it as simple as possible for people to get the results they want.

Most recently, we developed <u>Data-Driven Fasting</u>, which leverages your blood sugars to guide your fat-loss journey. The response and results have been phenomenal!

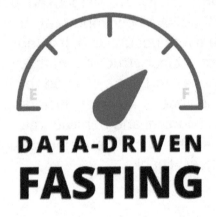

Ironically, after five years of trying to teach people to optimise what they eat, it seems that more people have more interest in not eating rather than learning how to eat well. However, the best results always occur when the two are paired together.

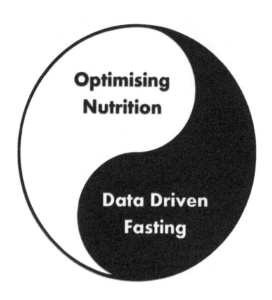

Why Am I Doing This?

This book aims to summarise the critical lessons and ah-ha moments that I have learned by writing hundreds of articles and working with thousands of people in the Macros Masterclass, Micros Masterclass, and the Data-Driven Fasting Challenge.

This is the book that I wish someone had handed to me when we started this journey. It includes:

- the most valuable lessons I've learned,
- things I once believed but have found were wrong and had to unlearn, and,
- simple action steps that will save you time and avoid confusion on your journey.

I would also like to remind you that I'm not a doctor. I'm an engineer. I just love numbers, graphs, and interpreting data.

I have devoted every available moment I have had over the past seven years or so to analysing, researching, and writing on nutrition and how we can fine-tune our food choices to align with our goals.

Please judge what you read on its merits and with an open mind. It's not always the most qualified people who have the 'Eureka' moments. More often, it's the people with personal motivation who come to a topic unblinkered by traditional education, who see things with fresh eyes.

Sadly, we often get it wrong when we try to apply our 'understanding' of science and biochemistry to human metabolism. We get caught up in a single magical mechanism and often miss the forest for the trees.

To get the most effective results with the least effort, we need to step back and look at the big picture to see if it aligns with reality for most people most of the time.

Who Is This Book For?

This book has been written for a range of different audiences.

- For people who have been following a 'keto' or low-carb way of eating and may not be seeing the results they hoped for:

    o This book will help them fine-tune their current eating methods to ensure they continue to move towards their goals.

- For people managing diabetes (either Type-1 or Type-2)

    o This book will help them understand how the food they eat affects their blood sugar and insulin and how to modify their diet to improve their results.

- For people interested in nutrition who just want to learn to eat better:

    o This book will give them fresh insights on how to view nutrition through the lens of Nutritional Optimisation.

What Is 'Optimal Metabolic Health' and Why Is It Important?

Health and nutrition can be confusing and overwhelming. There are lots of tests, technologies and things we can measure. However, you only need to apply the basics to move towards improved metabolic health and see results.

In this book, you will see the term 'optimal metabolic health' repeatedly. It's worth defining so you know what I'm trying to help you achieve.

As my good friend and Optimising Nutrition advisor Dr Ted Naiman likes to say, pretty much anything that makes you leaner and more robust makes you healthier. This is not merely a matter of being lighter, but instead having less body fat and more strength and lean muscle mass.

We're always looking for easy hacks and shortcuts to look and feel better. We can manage symptoms and markers with drugs and bio hacks, but they do not fix the problem and only give you better test results.

But managing symptoms and test results don't always make you healthier. Some common examples of symptom management include:

- injected (exogenous) insulin or avoidance of carbs to achieve stable blood sugars, so we look like we are lean and metabolically healthy,
- exogenous ketones or refined dietary fat to increase blood ketones, so we look like we are losing weight in an energy deficit,
- supplementation with vitamin D or melatonin so we look like we are young, healthy, sleep well, get adequate sun exposure, and have a well-calibrated circadian rhythm, and
- statins to reduce cholesterol, so our blood cholesterol levels conform to what we believe are healthy values, and so on.

We Are Overfed but Undernourished

These days, our food system is awash with cheap energy. We are overfed but undernourished. Thanks to fossil-fuel-based fertilisers, industrial agriculture and food processing, we have won the <u>war against hunger</u> and conquered <u>food security</u> issues we were trying to solve half a century ago.

Today, our modern food system makes it easier than ever to get energy. But getting the essential nutrients like vitamins, minerals, essential fatty acids, and amino acids that we really need to thrive are much harder to come by.

Nutrient-poor, low-satiety foods drive us to eat more than we need in search of the nutrients our bodies require for optimal health. Unfortunately, this quickly leads to energy toxicity or excessive amounts of energy in our bloodstream as high blood glucose, ketones, free fatty acids, and body fat. This energy toxicity, driven by our modern food environment, is the root cause of common modern diseases like obesity, Type-2 Diabetes, heart disease, autoimmunity and cancer.

To improve our metabolic health, we must make more informed food choices that will enable us to get the nutrients we need without consuming excess energy.

Rather than merely using more willpower, which usually leads to hunger, failure, guilt and rebound binging, we need to make smarter food choices that satisfy our bodies. Fundamentally, we need to find a way to give our bodies the nutrients they need without excess energy.

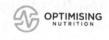

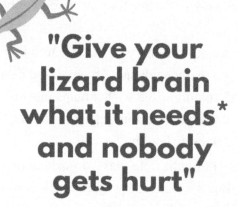

"Give your lizard brain what it needs* and nobody gets hurt"

*Seasonally appropriate & nutrient-dense food

Sadly, a dwindling minority of us are considered metabolically healthy. While we all don't need to identify as super-fit bodybuilders, most of us would benefit from having less fat and more strength and lean body mass.

It's not just about being lighter, but having less body fat and more muscle to ensure we are resilient as we age.

With just a tape measure, bioimpedance scale, and blood glucose meter, you can track your metabolic health at home and keep track of measurements like:

- body fat,
- lean mass and muscle,
- waist:height ratio, and
- fasting blood sugar.

You *May* Be a Unique Snowflake... But You're Probably Not

You *may* be a unique snowflake. However, I would be surprised if what you read here doesn't work for you if you apply the basic principles.

In this book, I offer my summary of the research that I have found most useful alongside my analysis of many large data sets. Together, this information shows what helps most people to manage their blood sugars, insulin, satiety, and body fat and move toward optimal metabolic health.

Over the years of riding the keto wave, I made numerous mistakes and believed in things espoused by 'gurus' that I later found didn't stack up. I would love it if you could avoid the potholes and dead ends on the road to nutritional enlightenment. I would also love it if the low-carb and keto communities listened, so they could continue to grow and help more people.

I have been banging this drum for a while now. The articles on Optimising Nutrition have had 4.2 million views from 2.3 million people worldwide.

Many have listened. Some have not. But I have tried. You will read here the highlights of my disagreements and opportunities for refinement of the theories that form the foundation of our current understanding of low-carb and keto science.

Unfortunately, most of the studies showing the benefits of keto and low-carb have been on epilepsy, cancer, or from people wanting to market some magical supplement. General health studies on a low-carb lifestyle have sadly been far and few.

This book is intended for people interested in using low-carb or keto to reach health goals of reversing diabetes, losing body fat, and optimising health and resiliency.

I hope my insights will provide some clarity to help people escape the tsunami of metabolic disease already crashing down upon us.

If we don't keep learning and moving forward, the consequences are ominous!

Common Misconceptions About 'Keto'

There have been many keto beliefs that have sprung up that we have later found to be incorrect. Over the past six years, I have spent a lot of time discussing these at length, analysing data to test these beliefs, and writing numerous blog posts sharing my learnings.

I put out a survey in the Optimising Nutrition Facebook Group to see what people thought I should cover in a book to address the most common areas of confusion.

As you can see from the survey results below, there was surprising enthusiasm and a long list of topics. These are some of the most common questions that have caused the most confusion and debate. I have endeavoured to address and add some clarity throughout the remainder of this book.

optimising nutrition

Added by Carol Dawn
Eat more fat to lose fat
56 votes

Added by you
Protein should be avoided because of gluconeogenesis
55 votes

Added by Carol Dawn
Energy balance is outdated science. Avoiding insulin spikes is how fat is lost.
48 votes

Added by you
Fat is a Free Food Because #insulin
27 votes

Added by you
"Optimal ketosis" is the goal. More ketones = better.
26 votes

Added by Chrestina Beebe Jones
ALL THE ABOVE!
22 votes

Added by you
You need extended fasting because autophagy
17 votes

Added by you
Carbs raise insulin, fat doesn't. So carbs are bad, fat is good.
16 votes

Added by Dave Bucci
You have to be in ketosis to burn fat
13 votes

Added by you
Fasting for longer is better
11 votes

Added by you
"Insulin Toxicity" is the primary enemy
10 votes

Added by Carol Dawn
Loose skin is repaired by autophagy
10 votes

Added by you
if in doubt, keep calm and keto on
9 votes

Added by you
Nutrient Density Doesn't Matter
8 votes

Added by you
Stable blood sugars will lead to fat loss
8 votes

A Brief History of Keto

Trends and fads come and go. Ideas rise in popularity when someone discovers something that works. A few people apply this initial idea and get great results.

In time, entrepreneurial people realise there is money to be made and scramble to sell things to make it 'easier' and 'more enjoyable'. Often, these marketers play fast and loose with the facts or don't even understand them to start with.

Later, once the benefits of the original insights become diluted or more people move beyond the initial stage where the idea magically works, the trend begins to die. Before long, something fresh rises to take its place as people search for a new, quick, and easy fix.

Over the years, there have been several iterations of low-carb and keto, each with its own unique emphasis, whether it be ketones, insulin, protein, fat, or something of the like.

Before we dive into dissecting the dogma and conflicting theories in nutrition, I thought it would be helpful to give you a quick tour of the different versions that have come and gone.

See if you can spot the common themes of successful lower-carb diets and the different emphasis over the years.

Banting

One of the earliest versions of low-carb was the 'Banting Diet', prescribed to English undertaker William Banting by Dr Harvey in 1862. Dr Harvey recommended a lower-carb, protein-focused, whole food diet that became super popular. Harvey had learned about the benefits of a low-carb diet to manage diabetes after attending lectures in Paris led by French physiologist Claude Bernard.

In 1864, Banting wrote a short booklet called *Letter on Corpulence, Addressed to the Public* as a testimonial of his success on Dr Harvey's advice. His daily diet consisted of four meals consisting of meat, greens, fruits, and dry wine. Banting's 'before and after' images are shown on the cover of two versions of his booklet, perhaps the first low-carb diet book in history.

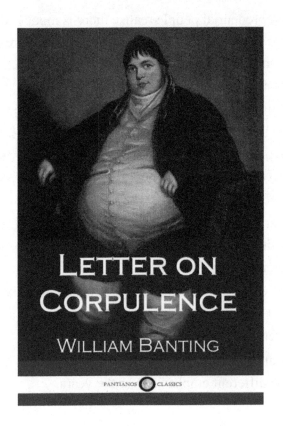

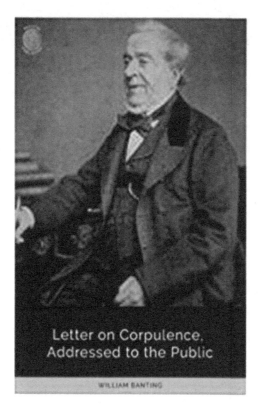

Letter on Corpulence, Addressed to the Public

WILLIAM BANTING

The term 'Banting' made a comeback in 2014 (as shown in the chart from Google Trends below), where it was spearheaded by South African Professor Tim Noakes. Noakes advocated a low-carb, high-fat version of the Banting diet and was careful not to overemphasise protein so that insulin remained low.

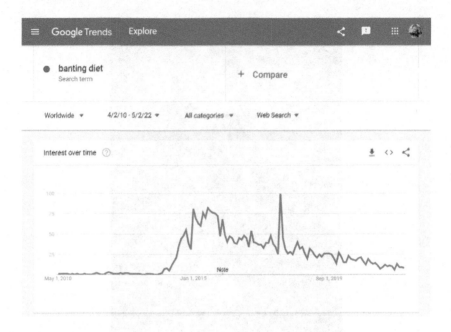

Dr Richard Bernstein

My family owes a massive debt of gratitude to the work of Dr Richard Bernstein and his followers. Dr Bernstein, who is thriving with Type-1 Diabetes at the age of 87, is an excellent example of how powerful carb reduction can be for people who are injecting insulin. Dr B (as his followers affectionally know him) also walks the talk in terms of maintaining strength to maximise insulin sensitivity and resilience.

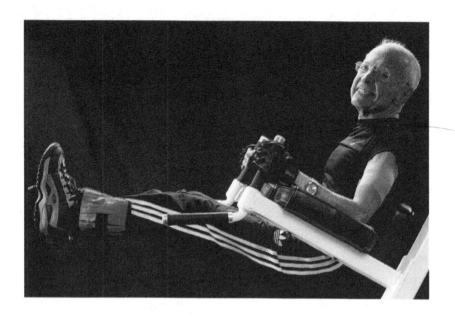

Bernstein, who has had Type-1 Diabetes since he was 12, was initially trained as an engineer. Through his wife, who was a doctor, he was able to obtain one of the first glucose meters in 1969 (pictured below).

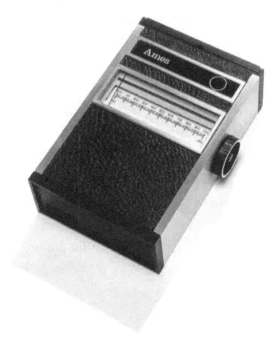

Bernstein, an avid self-experimenter, measured his blood sugars six times a day. Over time, he understood how much a certain amount of carbohydrate raised his blood glucose levels and how much insulin was required to lower them.

By reducing the carbohydrates in his diet, he stabilised his blood sugars and insulin doses. Bernstein's early learnings formed the basis of the basal/bolus insulin dosing calculations built into modern insulin pumps that many people with type-1 diabetes use today.

Bernstein initially published The Glucograf Method for Normalising Blood Sugar in 1981. At 45 years of age, he went to medical school and became a doctor to have his methods recognised. He later published:

- Dr Bernstein's Diabetes Low Carbohydrate Solution in 2005, and
- Dr Bernstein's Diabetes Solution: The Complete Guide to Achieving Normal Blood Sugars in 2011.

Bernstein's recommended diet is centred around protein to promote the growth of lean muscle mass. It also includes plenty of non-starchy veggies to ensure you get adequate micronutrients.

While many fear and try to minimise insulin, Dr Bernstein emphasises injecting sufficient insulin to maintain stable blood sugars after eating protein (protein requires about half as much insulin relative to carbohydrates over the first three hours).

Bernstein's approach to managing insulin and blood sugars revolves around 'The Law of Small Numbers'. That is, *large* inputs of refined carbohydrates require *large* doses of insulin.

Due to the numerous variables involved, it is incredibly hard, if not impossible, to precisely calculate the insulin dosage needed for large amounts of carbohydrates. As a result, large inputs of carbohydrates and insulin lead to large errors and the constant need for correction.

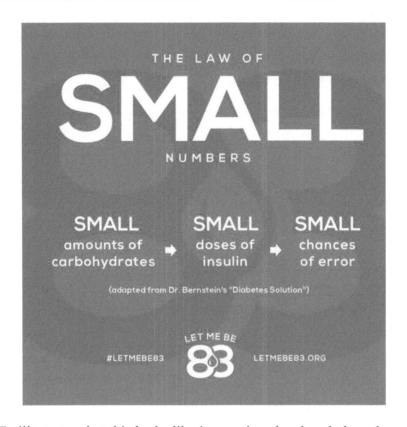

To illustrate what this looks like in practice, the chart below shows the blood sugars of someone with Type-1 Diabetes on a typical high-carb diet. Reducing the inputs of nutrient-poor processed carbohydrates reduces wild blood sugar swings and errors in insulin dosing.

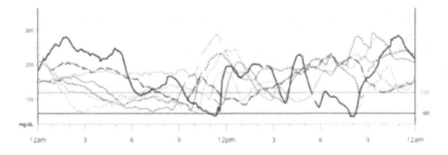

The next chart shows the blood sugar control that can be achieved once the inputs of processed carbohydrates are reduced. Once we minimise blood sugar variability, we can bring down the overall average blood sugar without the fear of low blood sugars (hypoglycemia).

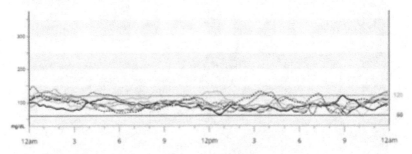

Monica and I were fortunate enough to be introduced to the Type One Grit Facebook Group in 2015. We became believers after seeing the fantastic results that could be achieved for people living with Type-1 Diabetes.

As we have applied these principles, the improvements in Moni's blood sugars, mood, energy, and weight have been life-changing. We are immensely grateful!

Bernstein's low-carbohydrate diet was initially opposed by the American Diabetes Association, which recommended a high-carbohydrate, low-fat diet for diabetics. In 2019, the American Diabetes Association changed its position to allow a low-carbohydrate diet as an acceptable option for diabetics. The UK NHS has also introduced a low-carbohydrate plan for diabetics and prediabetics.

Dr Robert Atkins

Interest in 'low-carb diets' peaked in popularity thanks to the work of Dr Robert Atkins, who published his carbohydrate-restricted diet for weight loss in 1972.

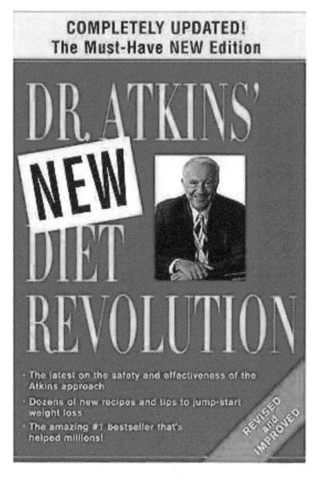

Dr Atkins' plan was focused on protein. While the definition of 'low-carb' can range from <u>20 to 150 grams of carbohydrates per day</u>, Atkins recommended an initial low-carb induction phase where less than 20 grams of carbs were consumed without emphasising extra dietary fat. This initial phase was followed by introducing some carbs from nuts and non-starchy vegetables, so long as the desired progress continued.

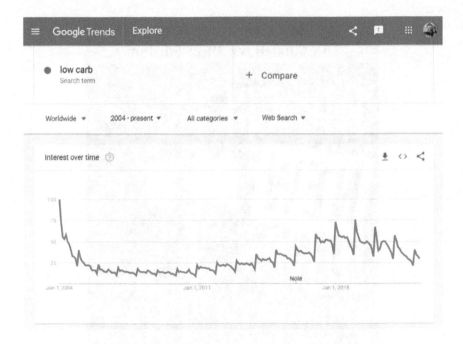

After Atkins died, interest in low-carb slumped to a low in 2008. Since then, low-carb has steadily grown in popularity—at least until January 2019—with each new wave of New Year's resolutions bringing a fresh surge of interest in how to shed the Christmas pounds.

Good Calories, Bad Calories

Investigative journalist Gary Taubes' 640-page tome *Good Calories, Bad Calories* (2007) created a comprehensive story around why carbs and insulin (rather than fat) could be behind the obesity epidemic.

Taubes highlighted the way hormones trigger appetite during growth spurts and pregnancy. He also showed the correlation between the introduction of sugar and refined grains to the native American diet (i.e., Pima Indians) and the subsequent growth in obesity.

After realising plenty of populations had been doing fine on a high-carb, low-fat diet, Taubes published The Case Against Sugar

(2016), painting sugar as the primary perpetrator of our metabolic woes.

These books have played important roles in cementing fears of insulin and carbohydrates into the psyche of low-carb and keto followers. Taubes' expansive narrative makes sense if you want to characterise one macronutrient as good vs bad. Good vs evil is imperative to any compelling story.

When you look at the increased carbohydrate intake between the 1960s and 2000, we can see that it correlates with the growth in obesity (at least up until 1999).

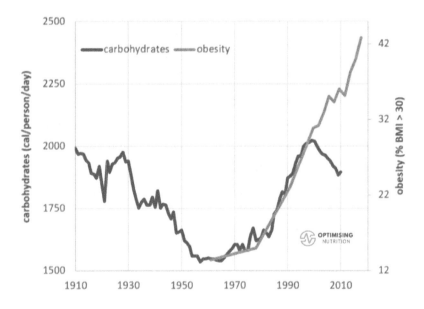

However, this 'single macronutrient' 'good vs bad' viewpoint neglects the fact that dietary fat, particularly from refined oils, has been on the rise in our food system for over a century.

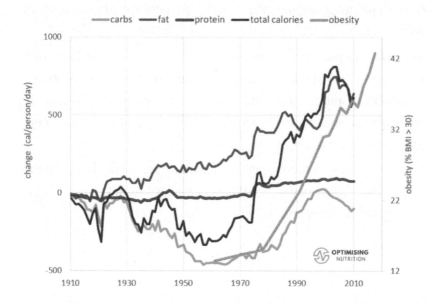

When we look at the change in energy from all three macronutrients, we can see the increase in obesity aligns with a change in total calories, mainly from fat and carbs (data for charts from United States Department of Agriculture Economic Research Service and the Centers for Disease Control).

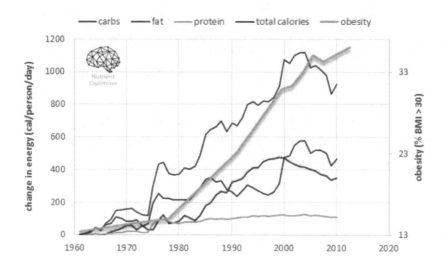

It's also worth noting that our sugar consumption has significantly *decreased* since artificial sweeteners replaced high fructose corn syrup (HFCS) in 1999. Although a constant supply of glucose and fructose (converted to fat in the liver) from sugar is far from optimal, this lack of correlation weakens the case against carbohydrates (and sugar) as the only culprit behind the diabesity epidemic.

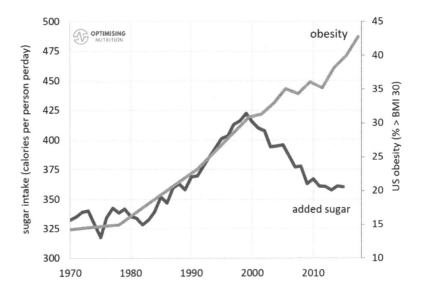

Taubes, along with Dr Peter Attia, formed the Nutritional Science Initiative (NuSI) to bring clarity to the fat vs carbs debate. Funded mainly by the Arnold Foundation, which provided $40 million to fund the research, NuSi instigated several studies to test the validity of the Carbohydrate-Insulin Hypothesis of Obesity. Admirably, NuSI chose lead researchers that weren't necessarily already proponents of the hypotheses it was trying to prove to avoid confirmation bias. One of these studies that we will be discussing later was the DIETFITs Study led by Professor Christopher Gardener at Stanford, which inconveniently showed a similar weight loss with either low carb or low fat.

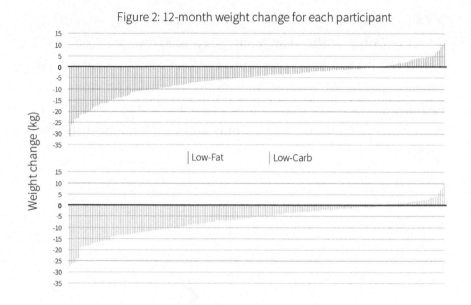

Figure 2: 12-month weight change for each participant

Another was the *Energy expenditure and body composition changes after an isocaloric ketogenic diet in overweight and obese men* led by Kevin Hall of the National Institutes of Health.

There has been plenty of debate around the interpretation of the study results, especially between Taubes and Hall. Since undertaking the NuSI study, Hall has led several studies that have cost in the order of $100 m to test the Carbohydrate-Insulin Model of Obesity and "to better understand how changes in fat vs carbs influence metabolic physiology, appetite regulation, and the role of insulin".

Unfortunately, it doesn't appear that many of the learnings from the studies that Taubes designed, arranged to fund for, and instigated have influenced his original narrative, which he reiterated in his recent book The Case for Keto.

Why Your Metabolism is Like the Stock Market

Before the 2008 Global Financial Crisis, I was fascinated by the art, science, and psychology of trading and spent a few years learning everything I could about the topic.

Before long, I realised there was no way I could know everything about the markets. Any news in the major press had already been factored into the price. Large investment funds have massive resources to understand market fundamentals that predict where the price will go in the future. Despite this, they often still get it wrong. While smaller traders can't match this firepower, they can jump on emerging trends. I spent a couple of years designing and testing my trading systems on all the data I could get my hands on.

Similarly, human metabolism is incredibly complex. We cannot understand all the moving parts and how they interact exactly. So, whenever we try to apply an overly simplistic theory, we fail. But we can stand back and look at inputs like macronutrients and micronutrients to understand how they influence the outcomes like energy intake.

We don't have to understand how it works or reduce it to one overly simplistic mechanism. Although it's always helpful to understand what we can about basic science, it's often more helpful to use the most powerful levers that make the most difference and follow in the footsteps of other people who have already attained the results we are looking for.

In retrospect, experience alongside my engineering background gave me the best foundation and training to approach quantified nutrition. It gave me the perspective to identify the levers that we can use to make the most significant difference to our health while discarding less useful theories that just create noise.

While it's great to do the research and try to understand how things work on a hormonal and biochemical level, you need to verify your theories with as much data as you can get your hands on to see if they help you achieve your goal in the real world.

Paleo

The Paleo Diet gained popularity in 2009, spearheaded by research biochemist Robb Wolf's book *The Paleo Solution* (2010). Interest in paleo peaked in January 2013, and paleo sadly never really escaped the wealthy, white, CrossFit scene to penetrate the mainstream.

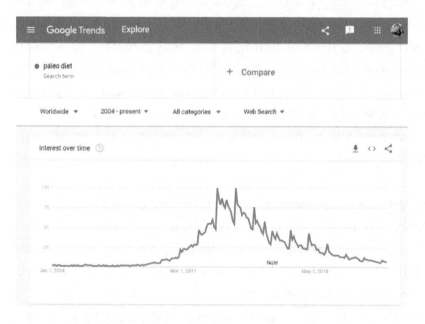

While not definitively low-carb, paleo tends to be lower in carbohydrates because it eliminates refined grains. The work of Dr Bernstein also influenced Wolf, and he also thrives on a lower-carb diet.

Wolf's second book, *Wired To Eat* (2017), included a 7-Day Carb Test where people are encouraged to check blood sugar after meals to understand if they need to reduce their carbohydrates to achieve healthy blood sugar levels.

Paleo seemed to flourish so long as people saw it as foods 'Grok the caveman' or your grandma would have recognised. However, once paleo comfort foods and products emerged, the diet lost its efficacy and quickly declined in popularity.

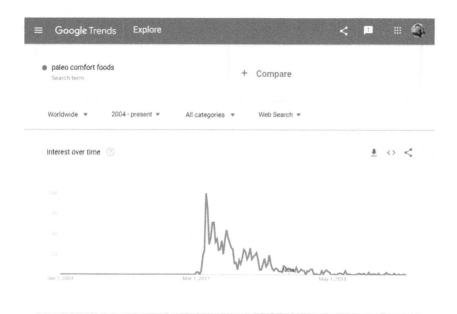

As proponents of the program soon discovered, if your goal is weight loss, it's not optimal to drown your sweet potato in butter or substitute processed foods with hyper-palatable, high-calorie concoctions of 'paleo approved' dates, honey, and coconut oil.

Carnivore

If low-carb is good, then Zero Carb must be better, right?

There has been an underground interest in Zero Carb for a while, but the 'carnivore diet' has overtaken Zero Carb over the past few years. While some people incorporate seafood and dairy, many simply advocate for 'eat meat, drink water'.

Amber L O'Hearn was one of the early carnivore advocates to manage her depression and bipolar and in an effort to manage her weight after low-carb. More recently, others have joined the carnivore tribe, like Dr Shawn Baker, author of *The Carnivore Diet* Mikhaila Peterson, Dr Paul Saladino, and the alternative health clinic Paleo Medicina that claims to use a paleo-carnivore diet to reverse chronic illness.

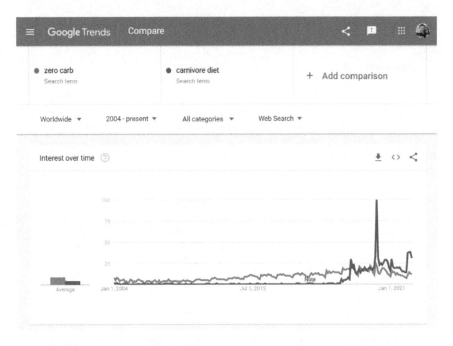

Many people with autoimmune issues have benefitted from eliminating plant foods in the short term and see great results. The carnivore diet provides plenty of bioavailable protein while eliminating the foods that people are most sensitive to. However, there are still plenty of arguments in carnivore circles over the appropriate balance between protein and fat from cross-pollinating the keto and carnivore communities.

Some proponents of the carnivore diet advocate a 'nose-to-tail' approach that emphasises organ meats to maximise nutrient density and compensate for some of the micronutrients that are harder to get without plant-based foods. However, many others abide religiously by the simple mantra of 'eat meat, drink water'.

While most people tend to thrive with more bioavailable protein (hence the success for so many), there may be limitations in obtaining optimal levels of some micronutrients on a diet comprised of just red meat.

For more discussion on carnivore, see:

- *The Carnivore Diet: Pros and Cons*
- *Optimising Dr Shawn Baker's Carnivore Diet From First Principles*
- *Optimising Dr Paul Saladino's Carnivore Diet*
- *Manifesto for Agnostic Nutrition*

Keto

The high-fat ketogenic diet initially began as a successful treatment for children with epilepsy in the 1920s. However, after the development of drugs to treat this terrible condition, the keto diet's popularity declined. However, keto outstripped low-carb, paleo, carnivore, and Banting combined.

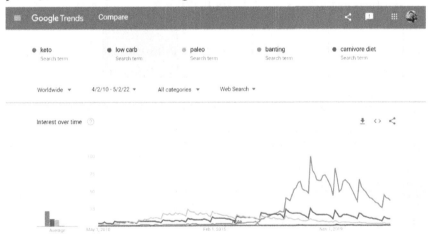

Google Trends indicates that searches for 'keto' peaked in January 2019 and have been trending downward since then. Only time will tell if it will power on or fade out because:

- too many people encounter the limitations of 'keto',
- people have a limited understanding of why it works, or
- followers don't understand how to tweak it to ensure their progress continues.

'Keto' means a lot of different things to the different people who have passionately embraced it and used it to describe their way of eating.

- For some, 'keto' means 5 per cent of total calories from carbs or less than 20 grams of carbohydrates.
- Others define 'keto' as any diet that produces a blood ketone level (i.e., beta-hydroxybutyrate) greater than 0.5 mmol/L.
- Still, others use keto to embrace fat as a 'free food' because it doesn't elicit a significant insulin response.

This lack of clear definition means that many people identify as 'keto' or 'keto-curious' despite their fundamental beliefs about what it is and how to do it differing significantly.

When we look at the history of various iterations of lower-carb diets that have worked well for people, the things that set keto apart from others are:

- a fear of 'excess protein', and
- a focus on achieving higher ketone levels and flat-line blood sugars.

As you will hopefully see, these differentiations may also be the fatal flaws of the keto movement.

My Journey Through Low-Carb and Keto Land

Eager to help my wife better manage her Type 1 Diabetes, I was an early adopter of keto, following all the podcasts and reading the latest research and blogs.

I enthusiastically devoured *Keto Clarity* when it finally came out in August 2014 and started adding butter, cream, cheese, and MCT oil to *everything* in pursuit of higher ketones.

I drank Dave Asprey's Bulletproof Coffee, believing it was the ultimate elixir of health. I even had a brief interlude with exogenous ketones.

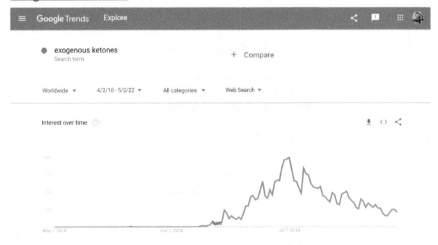

Much of the early keto movement was built on *The Art and Science of Low-Carbohydrate Living* (2011) and *The Art and Science of Low-Carb Performance* (2012) by Dr Stephen Phinney and Dr Jeff Volek. Both Phinney and Volek contributed to the *New Atkins New You* (2010) with *Cholesterol Clarity* and *Keto Clarity* co-author Dr Eric Westman.

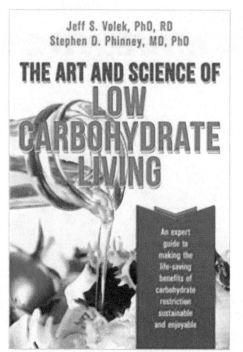

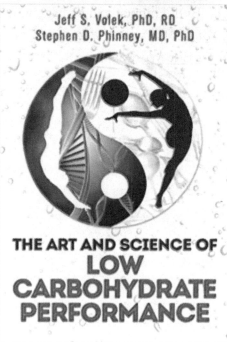

Why Keto Has Exploded (And Created So Much Division)

'Keto' first flourished as an underground movement rather than any government or official nutritional advice.

People following a keto diet saw themselves as rebels whose diet broke conventional rules. Now, there are seemingly <u>endless 'keto' groups</u> that each hold slightly different beliefs. This doesn't even begin to mention the numerous books, podcasts, and conferences with differing perspectives on the subject.

Keto thrived as an alternative to processed, 'healthy', grain-based nutrition dogma that is not working well for us. Sadly, the spiralling healthcare costs and decreased productivity from the <u>diabesity</u> epidemic threaten to bankrupt us in the foreseeable future.

Keto Has Its Limits

The 'keto' movement would not have exploded the way it has if it didn't prove to be beneficial for so many. There is no argument that countless people have greater <u>satiety</u> and better control over their blood sugars from 'keto' and low-carb diets.

There are plenty of critical keto reviews from 'outsiders' who have not lived and breathed either the diet or the community themselves. I *don't* want to add to that noise.

Keto has also had its fair share of detractors from mainstream dietary circles as well as the low-fat and plant-based camps. However, this debate has likely only fuelled the growth of the keto movement because controversy gets clicks.

My aim here is *not* to argue the value of low-carb and keto but rather to share the insights from my journey and data analysis. I hope we can continue to evolve our understanding of how it works to adapt and evolve to help more people who desperately need it! Any healthy, robust community needs to reflect and adapt as new insights come to light. But any group that refuses to change and becomes entrenched in dogma will not grow. Eventually, they will fade away and eventually die without refinement and adaptation.

While there are plenty of valuable insights that have been uncovered by biohackers, *N=1* self-experimenters, and gurus in the low-carb and keto communities, there are also plenty of half-truths that have flourished.

While harmless in small doses, much of the keto dogma can become dangerous if taken to the extreme—especially if you follow the 'keep calm and keto on' mantra while ignoring the sometimes-detrimental effects.

Hopefully, this book will add some nuance to these beliefs and help you get what you need long term.

Keto Lie #1: 'Optimal ketosis' is a goal. More ketones are better.

If keto is about anything, it's about ketones. However, one of the most confusing elements of keto is the concept of 'optimal ketosis'.

Many people believe that a higher beta-hydroxybutyrate, also known as β-hydroxybutyrate, BHB, or 'blood ketones', is better.

While this belief was based on the best information available, we now have better data as more people have followed a 'ketogenic diet' for many years. However, unfortunately, the recommendations haven't yet been updated.

To encourage people to strive for 'optimal ketosis' by simply boosting the level of consistently elevated ketones is unlikely to empower you to reach your goal of improved metabolic health.

Chasing higher ketones may even be dangerous as it encourages people to consume more nutrient-poor, high-calorie, low-satiety food that can cause energy toxicity and worsening metabolic health.

'Optimal Ketosis'... the Lie That Started the Keto Movement

In 2013, I watched a popular keto guru lose a massive amount of weight while tracking his ketones. It appeared that high ketone levels equated to fat loss. I wanted in!

So, I grabbed a blood ketone meter and started testing to see if I could get high ketones. Unfortunately, this made me fatter and more inflamed. The photo below is my work profile photo during my 'keto harder' phase.

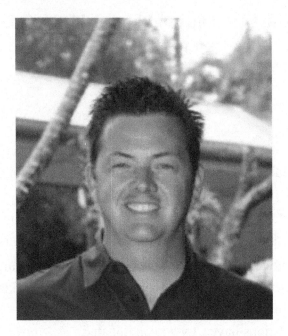

Much of the confusion around 'optimal ketosis' seems to be rooted in the 'optimal ketone zone' chart shown below, initially published in Phinney and Volek's *Art and Science of Low-Carbohydrate Living*.

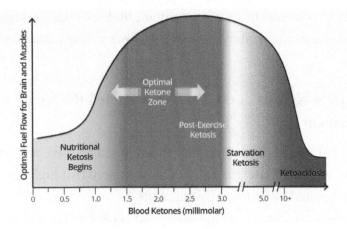

According to this chart, a 'ketogenic diet' generates blood ketone values greater than 0.5 mmol/L., also known as 'nutritional ketosis'. But, if you want 'optimal ketosis', you need to get your ketones above 1.5 mmol/L.

Some keto gurus have suggested that you should do whatever it takes to get your ketones into the 'optimal ketone zone' <u>by any means possible</u>. With ketones as the end goal, many recommend increasing butter, MCT oil, and exogenous ketone supplements if you want to lose weight and improve your health.

Many people advocating for this were part of a popular <u>multi-level marketing scheme</u> for exogenous ketone supplements. This may have clouded their judgement and recommendations.

I had the privilege of having Professor Steve Phinney (pictured below in our kitchen) stay at our place for a couple of days when he spoke at a <u>Low-Carb Down Under event in Brisbane</u> in 2016. During that time, I took the opportunity to quiz him about the basis of the 'optimal ketosis' chart.

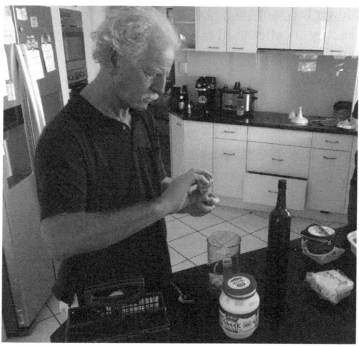

Steve told me the chart was based on the blood ketone levels of participants in two studies done in the 1980s. The first was with cyclists who had adapted to ketosis over six weeks. The second was a weight loss study where people were put on a ketogenic diet. In both cases, the critical thing to note is that 'optimal ketone levels' between 1.5 and 3.0 mmol/L were observed in *people who had recently transitioned to a lower-carb diet.*

However, as more people have 'gone keto', many people find their blood ketone levels continue to decrease after a few weeks or months on a 'ketogenic diet'.

We now know that ketone levels in our blood decrease as we become more metabolically healthy and better at burning ketones for fuel rather than having them back up in the bloodstream. In addition, it is now apparent that most people move beyond the 'keto-adaptation phase' after a few weeks or months as their bodies learn to use fat more efficiently.

Interestingly, the Inuit have a genetic adaptation that causes them to see lower levels of ketones on a high-fat diet. This is interesting because they are often used as an example of people who thrive on a very low-carb diet.

This progressive adaptation leaves many people faced with the decision to either:

- continue to add more refined fat from calorie-dense butter, MCT oil, and exogenous ketones to maintain elevated ketones in pursuit of 'optimal ketosis', or;
- reduce dietary fat to use body fat for energy, thus improving their metabolic health, reversing their diabetes, and reducing or obliterating obesity.

In an attempt to understand what was really happening, I compiled some data from my own testing and from friends and family who were also tracking their blood sugar and ketone values.

I wanted to understand what typical ketone levels were for people who reported that they had been following a reduced carbohydrate diet for more than a few weeks. Later, <u>Michel Lundell from Ketonix</u> shared an extensive set of anonymised data.

The chart below shows the sum of the blood sugar and ketones (i.e., total energy) from a broad range of people following a low-carb or ketogenic diet, represented as nearly 3000 data points. Blood ketones are shown in blue (on the bottom), while glucose is shown in orange (on the top).

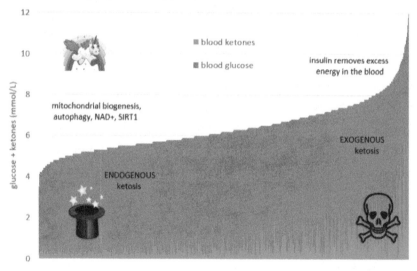

On the right-hand side of the chart, we have a high-energy state where both glucose and ketones are elevated simultaneously. While some people have high ketones and low blood glucose from endogenous ketosis, some people have high glucose and high ketones together. However, this is likely exogenous ketosis that has resulted from consuming high levels of dietary fat or ketone supplements.

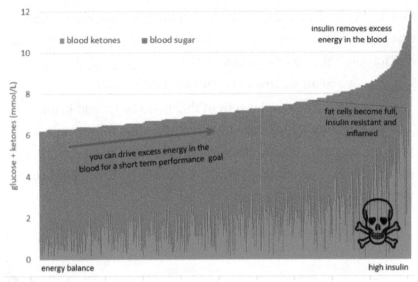

This high-energy situation is similar to someone with untreated Type-1 Diabetes, where high glucose and high ketone levels result from inadequate insulin production. Uncontrolled by adequate insulin, their stored energy flows into their bloodstream, and they see elevated levels of glucose, ketones, and free fatty acids.

Diabetic ketoacidosis (DKA) is a very dangerous state that usually only occurs in someone with uncontrolled Type 1 Diabetes. It is diagnosed when someone has glucose levels above 13.9 mmol/L or 250 mg/dL and significant ketones. This would equate to a quantity of *total energy* in the bloodstream of 11.5 mmol/L from glucose and ketones.

People with a healthy and functioning pancreas don't tend to see these extremely elevated levels. However, some people with glucose and ketone levels to the right of this chart are definitely on the spectrum of extreme energy toxicity.

While DKA and 'nutritional ketosis' are different, we need to stop and wonder whether having excessive amounts of energy in our bloodstream (i.e., energy toxicity) is desirable.

On the left-hand side of the chart, we see people with lower total energy in their bloodstream. We often refer to people who have plenty of storage available for glucose or fat as 'metabolically flexible'.

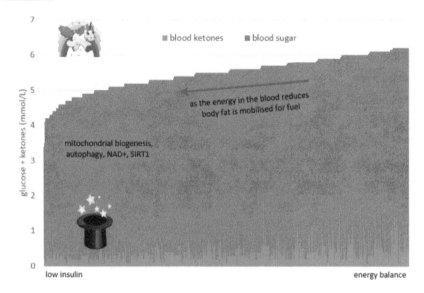

Because they store and use fuel efficiently, metabolically healthy people don't need large amounts of energy circulating in their bloodstream. Their fat stores are not overfilled, and they can easily hold fuel in storage and not in their bloodstream. As a result, their liver releases just enough energy into their blood when they need it to support their activity.

Some people come to keto to manage chronic conditions such as cancer, epilepsy, traumatic brain injury or dementia. These people appear to benefit from high blood ketones fuelling the brain when glucose cannot be used efficiently.

If you are trying to avoid muscle wastage from cancer cachexia or if you're trying to feed a growing child with epilepsy, an energy-dense, high-fat, low-satiety diet can help them gain weight while maintaining high levels of ketones.

People following a therapeutic ketogenic diet often load up with MCT oil and other added fats to achieve high ketone levels. Others target high levels of ketones with hopes of increased mental performance by loading up on exogenous ketones and glucose together to 'dual fuel' for elite athletic performance.

Although having sky-high levels of energy in your bloodstream may be beneficial if you're about to race in the Tour de France, chronically high energy from glucose *and* ketones simultaneously is not ideal if you are sedentary, trying to lose weight, or want to reverse your Type-2 Diabetes.

Most people do not require 'therapeutic ketosis', especially if weight loss or blood sugar control are their primary goals. These people need to optimise their diet to move towards a lower energy state that allows the stored energy on their body to be used.

The danger with trying to drive high levels of ketones by eating more fat is that it will lead to energy toxicity. This will drive up insulin and promote even more fat storage over the long term.

To summarise, for healthy weight maintenance, you want to see a total energy (from both glucose and BHB together) in your bloodstream less than 6 mmol/L. However, if you're losing weight, you may see this drift down towards 4.0 mmol/L.

How to Reverse Energy Toxicity

On the left-hand side of the total energy chart (i.e., glucose and ketones together), we have endogenous ketosis or ketones produced from utilising body fat for energy. By decreasing energy levels from both glucose and fat in your blood, your body draws on your fat stores to make up for the energy deficit. It will also use excess stored fat and old proteins in your liver, pancreas, brain, and other organs in a process known as autophagy.

This is a great place to be if you are trying to reduce your blood sugar, lose body fat, or improve your general metabolic health. As indicated by the little unicorn on the left of the charts, the real magic of ketosis happens when the ketones come from the fat on your body (endogenous ketosis) and not from energy sources like fat from outside your body (exogenous ketosis).

Reducing carbohydrates is beneficial *if* it moves you away from hyper-palatable processed foods that contain a hearty combination of carbs and fat. However, excessive levels of dietary fat will not be optimal if they lead you to increase your overall energy intake significantly.

Hopefully, you can now see that pursuing 'optimal' ketone levels as the primary end goal can be dangerous. If eating a 'ketogenic' diet causes you to add more nutrient-poor, low-satiety refined fat to your diet, it can *worsen* your insulin resistance and increase your body fat.

Dietary fat doesn't abruptly raise your insulin levels over the short term. However, as we'll see later in Keto Lie #5, it can still easily contribute to your body fat. In this sense, it can increase your insulin levels and insulin resistance.

The increased levels of energy in your blood (in the form of glucose, ketones and free fatty acids) will quickly lead to increased energy stored as fat in your body and increasing insulin to hold that fat in storage.

What Happens to Ketones on a 'Ketogenic Diet' Over the Long-Term?

It's interesting to see how the crowd-sourced ketone data in the charts above aligns with the Virta study one-year results (Phinney et al., 2017). This study aimed to get 262 participants with Type-2 Diabetes into nutritional ketosis to improve blood sugar management and reverse diabetes.

The distribution of BHB levels after 10 weeks of the Virta trial is shown in the chart below. While several people had higher ketone values, many people had values of less than 0.5 mmol/L even during the initial adaptation phase.

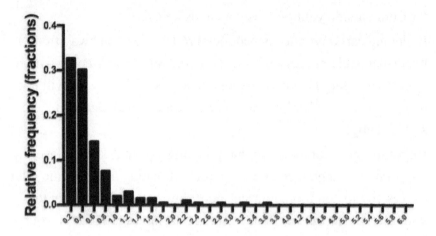

Despite consuming a 'ketogenic diet' under the supervision of the Virta Team, led by Steve Phinney, most study participants did not achieve ketone levels that qualified as 'nutritional ketosis' (BHB > 0.5 mmol/L) according to the 'optimal ketone zone' chart.

The following chart shows the average ketone levels of people participating in the Virta study over the first year (from *Effectiveness and Safety of a Novel Care Model for the Management of Type 2 Diabetes at 1 Year: An Open-Label, Non-Randomized, Controlled Study*).

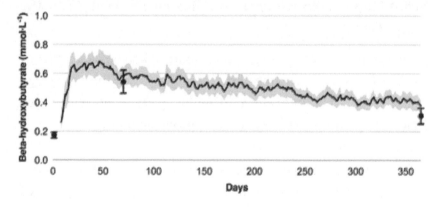

We see that blood ketone levels initially rose from 0.18 mmol/L at baseline to 0.6 mmol/L in the first few weeks. However, after a year, blood ketone values decreased to 0.27 mmol/L. This is well below the minimum threshold for nutritional ketosis of BHB > 0.5 mmol/L and far from the 'optimal ketone zone' of BHB > 1.5 mmol/L.

As shown in the chart below, blood ketone levels remained at 0.27 mmol/L after two years of Virta participants following a 'ketogenic diet' as people continued to lose weight and improve their diabetes (data from _Long-Term Effects of a Novel Continuous Remote Care Intervention Including Nutritional Ketosis for the Management of Type 2 Diabetes: A 2-Year Non-randomised Clinical Trial_).

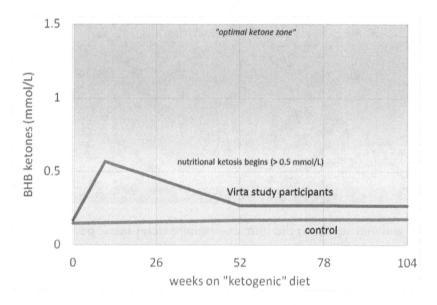

This data on the ketone levels of people adhering to a long-term keto diet was buried in the back of the paper and not discussed at all. If I had my way, the headline of the paper would have been, _'Blood ketone values are negligible after two years on a 'well-formulated ketogenic diet' as participants lost weight, reversed their diabetes and improved their metabolic health. So, why the hell are we still telling people to test ketones?'_

As shown in the chart below, we have seen a similar trend with ketones in our Nutritional Optimisation Masterclass. Blood ketones tend to rise for a couple of weeks when people focus on nutrient-dense, high satiety foods and meals and start to lose weight. But after a few weeks, however, blood ketone levels decreased as people continued to lose weight and lower their blood sugars.

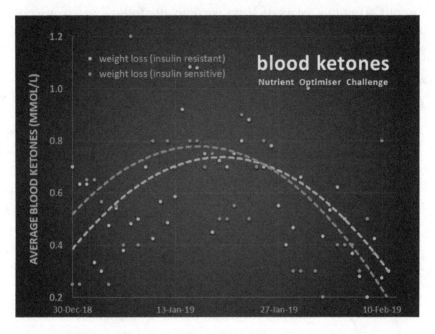

As you can see from the blue and orange trend lines, people who self-identified as insulin resistant saw their blood ketones rise more slowly. However, they stayed elevated for longer as weight loss continued.

People who are physically fit and with better markers of metabolic health (i.e., lower blood sugars, lower body fat, more lean mass and lower waist: height ratio) tend to have lower blood ketone levels. They also tend to have lower blood sugar levels, especially after following a low-carb or ketogenic diet for several weeks. Once your liver, muscles, and body fat are not filled to the brim with energy, it no longer overflows into the bloodstream.

Once your body uses up excess energy such as the glucose and ketones in your blood, it gets on with using the fat on your body.

Once you start to deplete the excess energy in your body, you are unlikely to see high energy levels backing up and overflowing into your blood.

What Are Optimal Ketone Levels for Fat Loss and Metabolic Health?

When it comes to defining 'optimal ketone levels', we need to be mindful of several things.

- While ketone levels can be elevated for a few weeks on a 'ketogenic diet', our bodies appear to adapt to use ketones more efficiently and (or) revert to using the citric acid cycle rather than ketosis to oxidise fat.
- Elevated ketone levels are associated with a high-energy state, fuelled by increased dietary fat or exogenous ketones. This may be beneficial for elite athletic performance or the management of epilepsy, Alzheimer's, and dementia.
- But if your goal is fat loss and improved metabolic health, we want a lower overall energy state where we generate ketones from body fat.

To clarify the topic of 'optimal ketosis', I prepared a chart that shows the range of blood ketones, blood sugar, and total energy you might expect to see when following a low-carb or ketogenic diet. The data is divided into five groups and is represented from the lowest to the highest total energy.

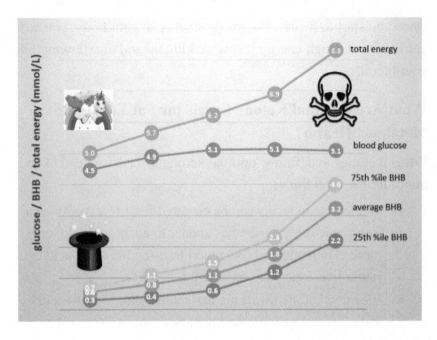

On the left, we have endogenous ketosis, where ketones are made from your body. On the right, we have exogenous ketosis, where ketones come from added dietary fat.

If you are part of the majority of people who want fat loss or improved metabolic health, you will want to move towards the left-hand side of this chart.

If you are on a ketogenic diet, relatively metabolically healthy and lean, and not overdoing the refined dietary fats, you will likely see BHB ketone values between 0.3 and 1.5 mmol/L.

Ketones will be higher if you fast, restrict calories, exercise, or consume more dietary fat. The level of ketones in your blood may be temporarily elevated when you start losing weight. However, it's important to remember that this is a side effect of weight loss and not the cause.

If your goal is exogenous ketosis, where ketones are produced primarily from the fat in your diet for the management of epilepsy, Parkinson's, or dementia, the 'optimal ketosis' values will be on the higher end of this range.

Remember that blood ketones will likely decrease over time as your metabolic health improves. As a result, many people conclude that blood ketones are not worth the expense, pain, or hassle.

Summary

- Your body produces ketones from your fat stores as an alternative fuel source for your brain and organs when there is no glucose, like when you go without food. This is known as *endogenous ketosis* because you are self-producing ketones in your liver from the fat on your body.
- When the supply of glucose and protein in our diet is reduced, your body can make ketones from the fat you eat. This is known as *exogenous ketosis*, or when the fuel for ketones is coming from outside the body.
- Most of the beneficial things we associate with ketosis like autophagy, lowered blood sugars, diabetes reversal, and fat loss occur when we use our body's energy stores because we are eating less. We can't 'bio hack' all these benefits by artificially elevating our blood ketone.
- We initially see higher beta-hydroxybutyrate (BHB) levels when people preliminarily switch to a low-carb or 'ketogenic diet'.
- Ketones tend to peak once we have drained excess glucose from the blood and glycogen stored liver.
- Ketone levels tend to decline afterwards as people continue to lose body fat and improve their metabolic health as they reduce the amount of stored energy.
- Any diet that stimulates fat loss is likely considered 'ketogenic' because you will be burning stored body fat. However, measurable blood ketones will likely decrease as we lose fat and improve our metabolic health over time.

- It's hard to make much sense of the number you see on your blood ketone meter to understand whether:

  o you are in the early stages of fat loss and starting to release stored energy into your bloodstream, or

  o you are overloading your system with excess energy that you are using inefficiently.

- Most people do not achieve the minimum ketone level to qualify for 'nutritional ketosis' (BHB > 0.5 mmol/L), let alone 'optimal ketosis' (i.e., BHB > 1.5 mmol/L) without adding excessive amounts of dietary fat.

- Merely adding more dietary fat will slow body fat loss, increase insulin levels throughout the day, and worsen metabolic health.

- While reducing dietary carbohydrates may help to stabilise blood sugars and improve satiety, tracking BHB is of limited use to help you optimise your diet or make more intelligent nutritional choices.

What Does This Mean for 'Keto'?

So, it seems that 'keto' has an identity problem.

- The most widely accepted definition of a 'ketogenic diet' is one that increases BHB above 0.5 mmol/L.

- However, we only see BHB ketones greater than 0.5 mmol/L in people who:

  o have recently transitioned to a low-carb or ketogenic diet,

  o are fasting for an extended period, or

  o are adding copious amounts of refined dietary fat or exogenous ketones to their diet.

- To maintain elevated ketone (BHB) levels, you must continue to increase the amount of nutrient-poor, low-satiety dietary fat, which can quickly lead to weight gain.

There are innumerable benefits from a diet that contains less processed carbohydrates. However, 'keto' has an identity problem by definition that is sadly causing many people to worsen their metabolic health, insulin resistance, obesity, and diabetes.

I would dearly love to see the 'optimal ketone chart' retracted. I believe it is potentially dangerous advice and has led many people, including myself, to worse metabolic health.

I published a blog post on this topic in July 2015 that has received nearly 383,638 views. I've also left plenty of comments on the Virta Facebook Page, where I shared my insights. Sadly, most of them were deleted.

I have spoken to Professor Steve Phinney and several other 'keto gurus' about this. But sadly, a large industry has built up around the strict 'keto' belief that elevated ketones are an end goal and the secret to optimal health.

Keto Lie #2: You Have to be 'in Ketosis' to Burn Fat.

Many people believe they need to be 'in ketosis' to burn fat. Because ketones rise when someone is burning body fat, they think fat loss is due to the ketones regardless of where they are coming from or need elevated ketones to lose weight. They then conclude that more ketosis is better, especially if there is body fat to burn.

While this belief helped sell keto-related products like recipe books and develop a cult-like following of people, it's simply not true.

Rather than simply believing that more ketones are better, it's critical to understand whether the ketones are:

- mainly coming from your body (endogenous ketosis) because you're in an energy deficit, or
- from drinking your third buttered coffee (exogenous ketosis).

What is Ketosis, and When Does It Occur?

Ketones are produced by the liver when fat is broken down. This fat can come either from your body or your diet.

While ketosis can be a *side effect* of fat loss, it is not the *cause* of fat loss, and it does not make your body burns its own energy stores.

Your body typically burns fat in the citric acid cycle, but it requires oxaloacetate from carbs or protein. Ketosis is simply an alternative metabolic pathway that your body can use when there is less dietary oxaloacetate from carbs or protein to burn fat via the citric acid cycle. When carbs and protein are low, the fat that can't be oxidised in the citric acid cycle is oxidised via ketosis.

The image below, created by certified nutrition specialist and author Amy Berger, demonstrates this graphically. On the right, we have the default process. On the left, we have ketosis, which occurs when there is inadequate oxaloacetate.

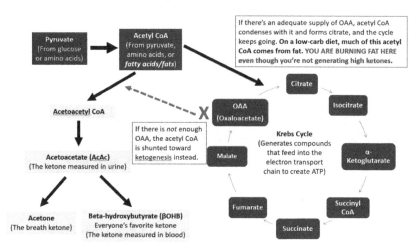

To quote my friend Mike Julian:

Ketones result anytime the citric acid cycle (TCA) in liver mitochondria encounters more acetyl-CoA than it can handle. This is a situation of relativity. However, as it can occur in two ways:

You can provide more acetyl-CoA to the liver TCA cycle by ingesting something like MCT oil or coconut oil. This surplus acetyl-CoA will exceed the TCA cycle's capacity, resulting in the balance being shunted towards the ketogenesis pathway. This will trigger ketogenesis even in the presence of carbohydrates.

But ketosis can also occur when we restrict carbohydrates or skip meals. In this case, the sharp decline in carbohydrates and decrease in liver glycogen creates a situation in which gluconeogenesis becomes prominent.

The very act of gluconeogenesis depletes the liver mitochondrial TCA cycle of oxaloacetate because it is donated to the process of gluconeogenesis. The TCA cycle can no longer operate at its previously higher capacity with less available oxaloacetate. Now, incoming acetyl-CoA will overwhelm the liver TCA cycle capacity more easily, resulting in the surplus acetyl-CoA being shunted off towards the ketogenesis pathway.

*In a low-carb setting, **ketogenesis is a by-product of gluconeogenesis**. Or, more broadly, ketogenesis is the result of the ratio of acetyl-CoA to the availability of oxaloacetate. Any time you create a situation where acetyl-CoA is higher than available oxaloacetate in the liver, the TCA cycle can facilitate ketogenesis.*

This backup metabolic pathway has helped humans survive many a famine. We see beneficial upregulations in mitochondrial biogenesis, sirtuins, autophagy, and the NAD+:NADH ratio when our energy levels are low. Our body goes into repair mode to ensure survival, and we switch over to burning body fat.

Many glorify ketosis as a magical state with many benefits. However, we often miss the fact that most benefits are NOT necessarily due to the ketones themselves but rather the energy deficit associated with endogenous ketosis when your body is using the fat on your body for energy.

What Does It Mean to Have High Blood Ketones?

Ketones take several different forms and roles in your body. As shown in the figure below, the energy that cannot be burned in the citric acid cycle enters as acetyl-CoA, where it is converted to ketones as acetoacetate.

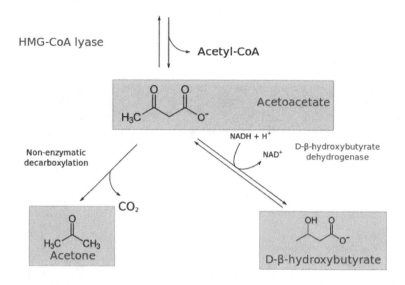

If your NADH:NAD+ ratio is high from excess stored energy in your body, ketones will be stored as BHB in your blood. Later, your body might have to convert BHB back to acetoacetate before it can be used for energy if required.

You can think of BHB as the storage and transport form of ketones in your body. The BHB ketones that you measure on your blood ketone meter tell you how much energy you have stored as ketones in your bloodstream. Unfortunately, the amount of BHB in your blood doesn't tell you whether you are using them for fuel or just filling your bloodstream with more energy.

We can liken the relationship of acetoacetate and BHB to glucose in the bloodstream and glycogen stored in the liver. Acetoacetate and glucose are burned in your body, while BHB and glycogen are the fuel storage forms that need to be converted back to the active forms used in your body.

What Are 'Peetones'?

Unfortunately, it's hard to measure acetoacetate levels, the active form of ketones, in your blood.

When someone is in the early stages of fasting or goes on a 'ketogenic diet', they can measure acetoacetate in their urine. These are sometimes referred to as 'peetones'.

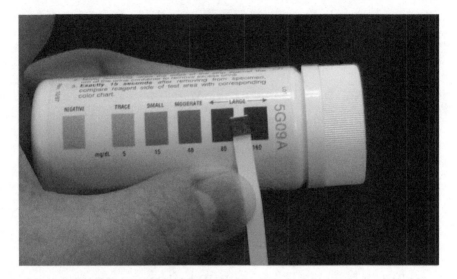

Most people deem acetoacetate in the urine to be a poor measure of ketosis because they tend to reduce to undetectable levels after a few days or weeks. People new to a 'ketogenic way of eating' often get confused and think they've done something wrong when they can no longer measure ketones in their urine.

However, the reduction in ketones may be because either:

- the body quickly adapts to using acetoacetate for energy, or
- with less oxaloacetate available and less reliance on ketosis to produce energy, we revert to burning fat more efficiently in the citric acid cycle.

Similar to high levels of BHB in the blood, spilling acetoacetate into the urine is not a sign that you are using ketones for energy. Instead, it indicates that you are making more ketones than your body can use.

It makes sense that our bodies would adapt to use all available energy rather than wasting it for too long.

Breath Acetone

While it is hard to measure the level of acetoacetate in your body, we can measure the acetone produced as a by-product when it oxidises to acetoacetate. This is commonly known as 'breath acetone', BrAce, or 'breath ketones'.

Measuring BHB has limited usefulness because we are measuring stored ketones. However, measuring breath acetone can help us determine whether we are using ketones (acetoacetate) for energy.

The Personal Fat Threshold

Some people think of diabetes as a disease of glucose intolerance. Hence, the solution is simply to avoid carbohydrates. But, thanks to Professor Roy Taylor's excellent work on the Personal Fat Threshold, we have come to understand that diabetes is related more to an inability to store excess energy from your diet as body fat.

Once your body fat stores become full, and you exceed your Personal Fat Threshold. Then, any extra energy from your diet is released into your bloodstream as high glucose levels, ketones, and free fatty acids are stored in your vital organs.

While most people become obese before developing full-blown Type 2 Diabetes, this is not always the case. For reasons that we don't fully understand that are likely related to genetics, race, inflammation, toxins and diet, some people can exceed their Personal Fat Threshold while still appearing relatively lean.

On the other extreme, some people can remain insulin-sensitive with healthy blood glucose levels even while putting on massive amounts of weight. The most insulin sensitive people can become very large before their bodies lose the ability to store excess energy from their diet as adipose tissue.

Once you can drain the excess energy from your body, your fat stores will be able to do their job efficiently. Excess energy will no longer back up and overflow into your blood. At this point, you will likely see lower levels of glucose, ketones, and free fatty acids in your blood.

Continuing to add more energy from dietary fat or <u>exogenous ketones</u> in the pursuit of higher ketones will only worsen the root cause of energy toxicity and commonly associated metabolic diseases.

The Glucose:Ketone Index (GKI)

We know from the previous chapter that lower glucose levels are a good thing, and ketones may be beneficial (depending on the context).

- In the absence of carbs or protein from the diet during starvation, BHB ketones can nourish the brain through endogenous ketosis, stay alert and find food.
- If we are managing conditions like Alzheimer's, epilepsy, or Parkinson's, therapeutic ketosis via exogenous ketosis also appears to be beneficial.
- High ketones are not desirable if they are also accompanied by high blood glucose levels or free fatty acids. You are merely driving a high energy state in your body with lots of extra fuel.

One way to ensure we are not overloading our system with excess energy from our diet is to ensure that higher ketone levels are accompanied by lower glucose levels.

Professor Thomas Seyfried developed the glucose: ketone index (GKI) (see *The Glucose Ketone Index Calculator: A Simple Tool to Assess Therapeutic Efficacy for Metabolic Management of Brain Cancer*).

<u>Seyfried advocates fasting for cancer patients</u> and uses the GKI to track their metabolic health during fasting. As discussed in <u>Optimal Nutrition for Cancer Management</u>, excess glucose and the

surplus of energy that is associated with obesity appear to drive cancer growth.

If insulin levels are not excessive, we would see higher BHB ketones during a fasting period as glucose levels decrease and ketone levels rise to make up for the energy deficit.

To understand what the GKI might look like in practice, I plotted more than 1,200 blood glucose versus ketone values using data supplied by Michel Lundell of Ketonix.

These values are divided into five groups based on their GKI value. If you were fasting, a lower GKI would be better; your blood glucose levels would be low, and your ketones would rise to supply the fuel necessary for your brain and vital organs.

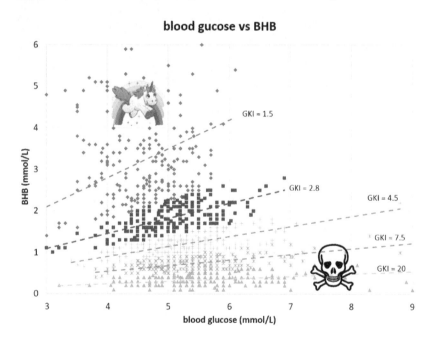

blood gucose vs BHB

The people with the worst metabolic health are represented by the green dots at the bottom of the chart where GKI = 20. These people have high blood glucose levels and low ketones, and their glucose values are 20 times that of their ketone values.

Most of the time, people will not get GKI values under 2.0 until they fast for a few days. The chart below shows what you could expect if you fasted for seven days based on my data combined with several others who tested their ketones and glucose during an extended fast.

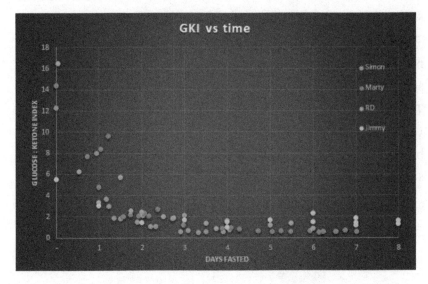

However, the problem with the GKI again comes when people confuse exogenous ketones (from *outside* the body) and endogenous ketones (from *within* your body) or think they are equivalent.

Lately, the GKI has sparked interest in Ketoland, with many people chasing a lower GKI as a badge of honour. Rather than monitoring long-term fasting as designed, more people are combining fasting with high-fat eating to get lower GKI values.

Sadly, this is unlikely to lead to optimal body composition over the long term. Adding more low-satiety, nutrient-poor refined fats to keep GKI values low will exacerbate metabolic issues by driving energy toxicity.

The Glucose:Acetone Index

If you wanted to check if you were burning rather than storing fat using ketones, breath acetone (BrACe) might be a more useful measure of beneficial ketosis.

When the storage form of ketones BHB is converted to acetoacetate for energy, acetone is released as a by-product and can be measured by breath.

Acetone is a vapour similar to nail polish fumes that is released from acetoacetate. If you are releasing a high level of breath acetone, you may experience fruity-smelling breath or a metallic taste in your mouth.

You can measure BrAce to understand if you are using ketones rather than just storing them. Many people now seem to be showing more interest in breath acetone after noticing that it yields better outcomes in patients using ketosis therapeutically.

I plotted 2500 glucose and breath ketone readings in the chart below to better understand the relationship between breath acetone and blood glucose.

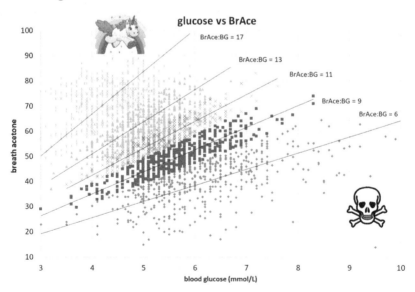

You can see from this chart there is a similar relationship between glucose and breath ketones as with blood ketones, but there is less scatter than with the GKI chart. Blood glucose and breath acetone are correlated more closely than blood ketones.

It's hard to have high breath acetone with high blood glucose levels. You can't manipulate the system by forcing in more and more dietary fat or exogenous ketones the same way you can with BHB.

The optimal situation is to have lower blood glucose levels with a significant amount of breath acetone in your system. This would indicate that you are producing ketones without consuming excess energy.

You'll probably fall in the purple or green areas on the chart towards the top left if you have good metabolic health. If you reach a therapeutic level of ketosis or fast for extended periods, you will ideally fall in the upper left area that is green or light blue, with low glucose and high breath ketones.

Different breath ketone meters, unfortunately, use different units for BrAce, so it's hard to standardise a good versus bad glucose:BrAce ratio. However, if you wanted to track glucose and breath acetone simultaneously, you would want to see the ratio increase over time. This would indicate that your glucose is dropping and that you are effectively oxidising ketones.

Should You Measure Ketones?

If you require therapeutic ketosis to manage conditions such as epilepsy, Alzheimer's, or dementia, then it may be helpful to monitor ketones.

Given that BHB ketones are more a measure of the energy stored in your body and BrAce is more a measure of how well you're using ketones for energy, BrAce may better indicate if you are utilising ketones for energy rather than storing them.

If you want to track your ketones and glucose, the glucose to breath acetone ratio will be the most useful thing you can measure. Over time, you want to see your breath acetone divided by your glucose increase as your metabolic health improves.

However, if you do not require therapeutic ketosis, simply monitoring glucose, weight, waist, and perhaps body fat will give you most of the information you require to ensure you are moving in the right direction.

Is There a Specific Number That Indicates I Am in 'Fat-Burning Mode'?

The concept of a single magic number that indicates you are burning fat or in 'fat-burning mode' is alluring as measuring blood ketones does not tell you whether that fat is coming from the high-fat food you are eating or your body.

If your goal is body fat loss and improved metabolic health, tracking your blood glucose before eating is likely more useful. The best way to manage your pre-meal glucose value is to simply wait a bit longer to eat until your body has used up more of the glucose in your system. As your premeal blood glucose levels reduce, your body will progressively turn to burn more fat, particularly at rest.

Summary

- You don't need to be 'in ketosis' or have elevated ketone levels to burn fat from your diet or body.
- Ketosis is an alternative pathway that your body uses to burn fat in the citric acid cycle when you don't have enough carbs and protein available for energy production.
- When you eat enough carbohydrates or protein, you will be burning fat in the default citric acid cycle.
- If you eat a satiating diet that leads to an energy deficit with adequate protein, you may have lower ketones, but you will still be burning fat.
- Measuring blood ketones is of limited use to guide your dietary choices because it is hard to know whether the fat is

coming from your body or your food.

- Low glucose with higher ketones (especially breath ketones) may be more beneficial to track improved metabolic health via helpful markers like the glucose: acetone index.
- Waking glucose and your waist to height ratio is an excellent indicator of insulin resistance.
- Monitoring blood sugar before you eat is more valuable to guide meal timing and ensure you are moving towards improved metabolic health.

Keto Lie #3: You Should Eat More Fat to Burn More Body Fat.

O ne of the most common responses to a weight-loss stall in keto groups is to 'eat more fat to get your ketones higher and burn more fat'.

This lie is seductive because it is partially true and delicious! High-fat foods are highly palatable and provide a dopamine hit that makes us feel great and gives us a quick energy rush.

However, it's important to understand that burning dietary fat or body fat can generate higher ketone levels. This distinction is vital if you are going to achieve your long-term goals.

Has Reducing Fat Helped Us?

Like all macronutrients, dietary fat is a controversial and divisive topic. And, as with many popular myths, there is an element of truth to the belief that eating fat will enable us to burn fat.

Understandably, many people have swung hard to one extreme or the other. Since the 1977 Dietary Guidelines release, we've been told to avoid fat, particularly saturated fat and cholesterol. However, despite obediently reducing these 'bad foods', the obesity epidemic has marched on unabated.

The charts below show that we have obediently reduced the percentage of energy in our diet from both saturated fat and cholesterol per the guided recommendations (data from the United States Department of Agriculture Economic Research Service and the Centers for Disease Control). This has been achieved by eating fewer animal products and more high-profit margin refined grains, sugars, and seed oils from large-scale agriculture.

However, reducing the amount of saturated fat and cholesterol in our diet has not helped us reverse the runaway diabesity epidemic, as the charts below show. If you were cynical, you might think that the fear of cholesterol and saturated fat was just a brilliant marketing campaign to sell more high-profit margin products made from nutrient-poor, low-satiety refined grains, sugars, and seed oils.

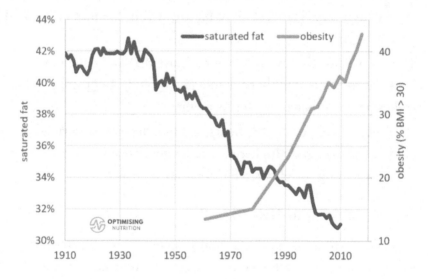

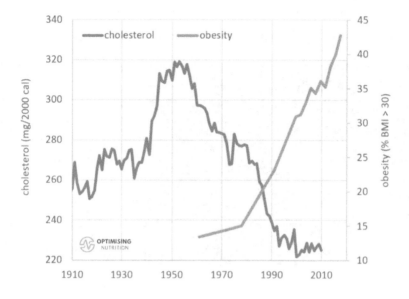

When we were told that we could eat fat and get skinny, many people jumped on board to swing to the other extreme believing that fat could do no wrong. However, a recurring theme of Optimising Nutrition is that the optimal is rarely found at extremes, especially when it comes to our food.

Response To Anything

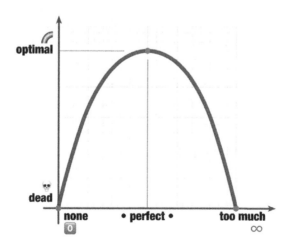

We love thinking in terms of 'ON vs OFF', 'black vs white', 'right vs wrong', and 'us vs them'. But it's rarely that simple!

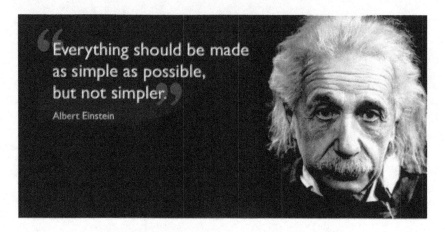

The DIETFITS Study

So, does replacing carbs with fat help you to eat less and lose weight?

Let's see what the data tells us.

In partnership with Gary Taubes and Peter Attia's Nutritional Science Initiative, Stanford University carried out a ground breaking, year-long major study with more than 609 participants (*Effect of Low-Fat vs Low-Carbohydrate Diet on 12-Month Weight Loss in Overweight Adults and the Association With Genotype Pattern or Insulin Secretion: The DIETFITS Randomized Clinical Trial*).

As shown in the charts below, the study found that participants following either a low-fat or low-carb diet achieved similar weight loss and improvements in metabolic health, regardless of genetics, insulin levels, or blood sugars.

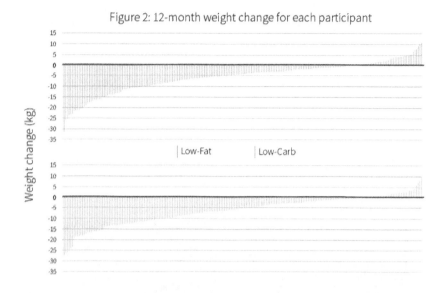

Figure 2: 12-month weight change for each participant

Researchers initially encouraged participants to pursue a diet as low in carbs or fat as they could achieve. They then asked them to back off to a level that they felt was sustainable.

The key observations from the Stanford DIETFITS study were as follows:

- Following either a low-carb or low-fat diet can help reduce hyper-palatable, highly processed junk food that typically causes us to eat more than we need.

- Over time, most people gravitate back to hyper-palatable junk food, which is typically a combination of nutrient-poor fats and carbs.

- The people who changed their diet QUALITY had the most significant long-term success. These people experienced increased satiety and no longer felt like slaves to their appetites.

Lead researcher Professor Chris Gardner stated that defining diet quality to achieve satiety rather than pursuing a magic macronutrient ratio is the next exciting nutritional science frontier. Empowering people living in the real world to gain control of their appetite will free them from weighing and measuring everything they eat and continually having to fight their hunger.

Plant-Based Low-Fat vs 'Well-Formulated Ketogenic Diet'

In a similar vein to the DIETFITS study, Kevin Hall's NIH group recently published *A plant-based, low-fat diet decreases ad libitum energy intake compared to an animal-based, ketogenic diet: An inpatient randomised controlled trial*.

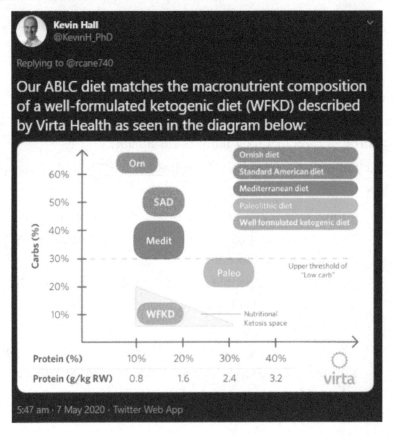

Their goal was to compare macronutrient extremes by comparing results between a 75% carbohydrate (PBLF = plant-based low-fat) diet and a 75% fat 'well-formulated ketogenic diet' (ABLC = animal-based low-carb).

There is no argument that the people on the keto diet were in ketosis. BHB levels reached 2.0 mmol/L towards the end of the two weeks in the low-carb population (ABLC = red line).

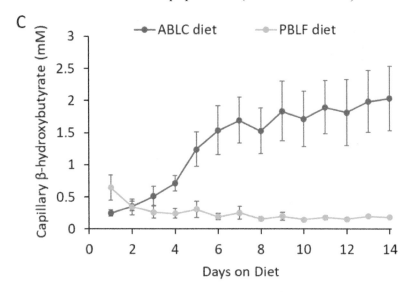

Blood glucose levels were more stable and a little lower on the low-carb diet (ABLC = red bars). HbA1c, average glucose, and insulin levels improved on both diets, but slightly more on the low-carb (ABLC = red bars).

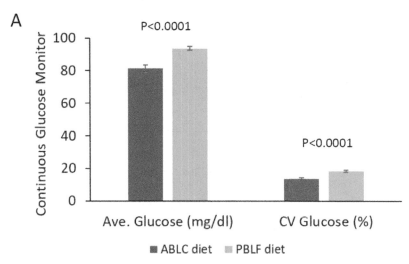

There was a flatter and smaller blood sugar response on the low-carb diet (ABLC = red line) than on the low-fat diet (PBLF = green line).

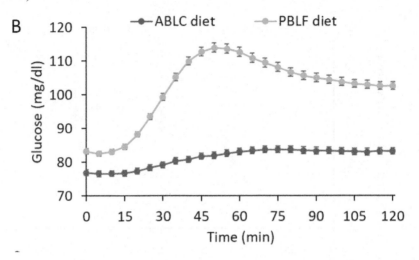

However, as per the study headline, participants averaged far fewer calories on the low-fat diet (PBLF = green line)!

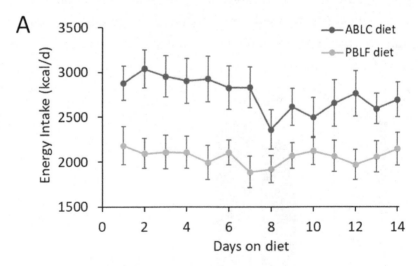

Participants on the low-carb diet lost more weight than on the high-carb diet, although the difference between them was not great enough to be statistically significant.

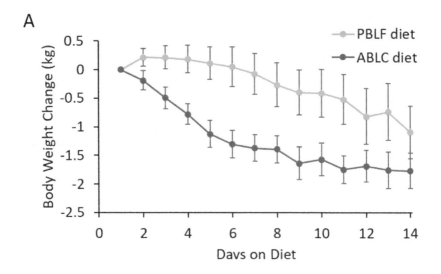

Weight loss on the keto approach was more water weight, whereas those on the low-fat diet lost slightly more body fat. This is because of the water weight retained with the glycogen in the liver. *Note: every gram of glycogen is stored with 4 grams of water, resulting in a more significant initial weight loss as blood sugar drops.*

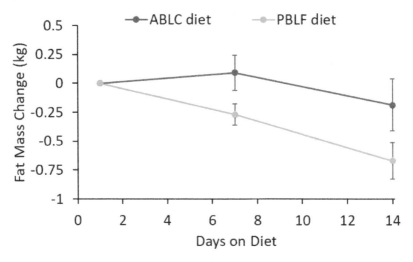

While the Twitterverse lit up with plant-based and keto camps, with each claiming their respective team had won, the reality is the results were pretty much even. Similar to the DIETFITS study, everyone lost weight when they moved away from hyper-palatable processed foods that typically combine fat and carbs.

Why Does Low-Carb Work?

If it's not about carbs or fat, why do we still have an obesity epidemic?

It seems we need to go beyond thinking in terms of carbs vs fat. Unfortunately, neither study tested a control arm in the middle. I would have loved to see what would have happened if they compared it with a hybrid that contained a similar blend of carbs and fat together.

Fortunately, our satiety analysis helps to fill in these gaps. The chart below is from our analysis of 587,187 days of food logging. The vertical axis shows users' actual calorie intakes entered into MyFitnessPal divided by their target calorie intake.

A value toward the bottom means they consumed less than their goal and *vice versa*. We divided the days of data up based on their carbohydrate intake (shown on the horizontal axis).

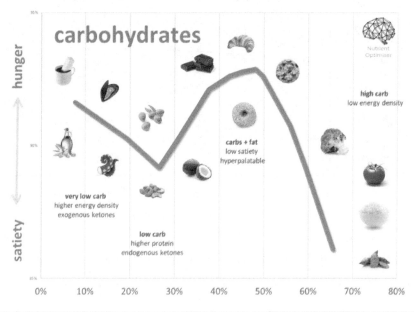

The green line indicates that we tend to eat a greater quantity of food when that food combines fat and carbs, like doughnuts and croissants (i.e., 40-50% carbs, with the rest of the energy from fat).

As we move toward the left, reducing dietary carbohydrates tends to help us eat less, but only up to a point. The best satiety outcome occurs when carbohydrates make up about 25% of total calories.

To the right, we see that it is tough to over-consume foods like broccoli, plain rice, and plain potato that have a very high carbohydrate content and are very low-fat.

Why We Love Carb and Fat Combo Foods

Dopamine is a neurotransmitter that makes us feel good. It also reinforces generally beneficial behaviours and helps us form habits that ensure our survival.

Some examples of things that produce dopamine include: eating food that contains energy tastes great because it has the nutrients we need, learning something new, sex, and other similar actions.

The combination of fat plus carbs provides the biggest dopamine hit because it enables us to fill our fat and glucose storage tanks simultaneously. This observation aligns with a 2018 study in Cell Metabolism that showed fat and carb foods give us a 'supra-additive' dopamine reward.

Clinical and Translational Report

Cell Metabolism

Supra-Additive Effects of Combining Fat and Carbohydrate on Food Reward

Graphical Abstract

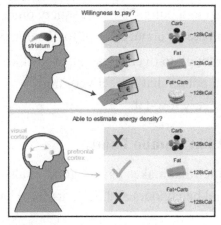

Authors

Alexandra G. DiFeliceantonio,
Géraldine Coppin, Lionel Rigoux,
Sharmili Edwin Thanarajah,
Alain Dagher, Marc Tittgemeyer,
Dana M. Small

Correspondence

dana.small@yale.edu

In Brief

DiFeliceantonio et al. show that foods containing fat and carbohydrate are more reinforcing than equicaloric foods containing primarily fat or carbohydrate. This effect is independent of liking and is reflected by supra-additive responses in the striatum during food valuation. This may be one mechanism driving overconsumption of high-fat/-carbohydrate processed foods.

Highlights

- Fat and carbohydrate interact to potentiate reward independently of liking

- This is reflected in supra-additive responses in the striatum during food valuation

- Participants are able to estimate energy density from fat, but not carbohydrate

- Accurate estimation of energy density recruits a prefrontal-fusiform gyrus circuit

This relationship between energy intake and combining macronutrients also aligns with *Body fat and the metabolic control of food intake* (Friedman 1990).

(high fat) + (high carb) + (high energy) = hyperphagia

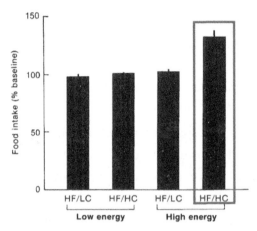

Fig. 4. *Effect of diet composition and energy density on energy intake in rats.* Data are changes in daily intake averaged over a 4 week period relative to a baseline period when rats were fed a standard laboratory diet (Purina Chow). HF/LC, high-fat/low-carbohydrate diet; HF/HC, high-fat/high-carbohydrate diet; low energy = 3.3 kcal/g (13.8 kJ/g); high energy = 4.7 kcal/g (19.7 kJ/g). Values are means ± s.e.m. of 9 rats per group.

In this study, *ad libitum* feeding (as much as they wanted) was used in rats. Researchers were able to conclude that 'the signal for overfeeding originates in the liver when both fatty acids and glucose are available for oxidation'.

Our brain is programmed to seek out fat and carb combo foods and find them incredibly delicious because they are effective at getting us calories quickly and storing fat! These energy-dense foods are rare in nature other than in autumn to help animals prepare for winter. However, the fat and carb formula is the basis for most modern processed foods.

Food manufacturers and recipe book creators have perfected the art of combining refined grains and sugars with processed oils that make food palatable. Why? So, you eat more. These foods also typically contain added flavourings and colourings to trick our brains into thinking these foods contain the nutrients we require (but they don't).

> *The food problem is a flavour problem. For half a century, we've been making the stuff people should eat—fruits, vegetables, whole grains, unprocessed meats— incrementally less delicious. Meanwhile, we've been making the food people shouldn't eat, like chips, fast food, soft drinks, and crackers, taste even more exciting. The result is exactly what you'd expect.'*
> Mark Schatzker, The Dorito Effect: The Surprising New Truth About Food and Flavour

Many people report a spontaneous reduction in appetite when they reduce processed carbs in their diet. However, it appears that the main benefit of a low-carb, high-fat diet comes from lowering carbohydrates. This change moves us away from hyper-palatable fat and carb foods—NOT the focus of eating more fat!

The frequency distribution (blue bars) shown in the carbohydrate vs satiety chart below demonstrates that most people gravitate to low-<u>satiety</u> foods that contain around 40% of their energy from carbs and a similar amount from fat.

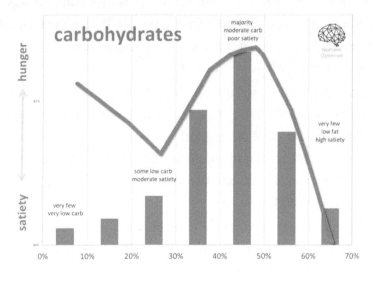

To the right of the chart, we see that not many people manage to eat very high-carb, low-fat diets that can lead to much lower energy intake. However, groups of people follow a low-fat, whole-food, plant-based diet that demonstrates this, although the profile of bioavailable micronutrients may be less than optimal.

While it's hard to get fat on a diet consisting only of fruit and vegetables with no added oil, it also requires a significant amount of time to prepare and consume. Thus, most people opt for convenience and add refined oils to ensure they get the energy they crave.

When we move to the left, we see that a lower-carb diet with 20–30%from carbs provides an improved satiety response and a lower *ad libitum* calorie intake. However, moving to an even lower carb intake is not necessarily better.

High-Fat Keto Works... Until It Doesn't. But Then What?

Many people find that reducing processed carbs and not fearing fat in the early days of a low-carb or keto diet is helpful. Their blood sugars stabilise, and they lose a lot of water weight.

As noted earlier, you store 4 grams of water for every gram of glycogen in the liver and muscles. As a result, you also lose a significant amount of water and weight on the scale as you deplete glucose.

If you slash all your carbs and don't replace them with fat, you'll likely feel overly hungry, and you won't stick with your diet. Instead, it can be wise to just reduce carbs without initially focusing on cutting fat.

Low-carb foods also tend to contain more bioavailable protein, which boosts satiety so that people feel fuller. People can then control their weight without tracking their food. They fall in love with their effortless new weight loss and believe all the benefits are from the fat they're eating and not reducing carbs or increased protein. However, a low-carb, high-fat diet often works for a while... until it doesn't.

Once you've gained the satiety benefits of more bioavailable protein and moved away from the hyper-palatable carb and fat danger zone, the hardest but most necessary step is likely to start dialling back dietary fat, too.

Like stealing a new toy from a baby, it can be hard to reduce dietary fat if we've been told—and subsequently believed—that we could have as much of it as we wanted. Sadly, it may be necessary if we're going to continue to make progress in terms of fat loss and diabetes reversal.

Tammy von Keisenberg
This has worked brilliantly for me. I was going around in circles, losing the same kg over and over again. Increasing, almost doubling, my protein and simultaneously lowering my fat intake, has seen me lose 19kgs since January. Who knew it was this easy. 😌

Like · Reply · 6 h   ⚙⚙ 2

For continued weight loss, we need to think in terms of eating to get the nutrients like protein, vitamins, and minerals we require from the food we eat while allowing excess stored energy to be used.

Is it Better to Reduce Carbs or Fat?

The chart below shows the satiety response to fat and non-fibre carbohydrates on the same chart showing that we achieve a similar response to reducing either fat or carbohydrates. Moving from 40-50% to 10-20% non-fibre carbs has a similar impact on how much you will eat as moving from 80% fat to 35% fat.

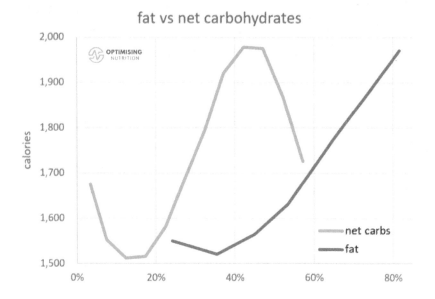

When we look at the satiety response to all the macronutrients together, we see that reducing the energy from fat and carbs, which increases our percentage of energy from protein, has a much more significant impact than focusing on carbs or fats alone.

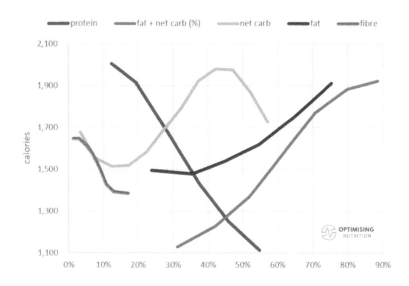

As we will see in the next chapter, it's not carbs or fat but rather the percentage of protein in our diet that is the most significant lever on our satiety and how much we will eat.

Summary

- Reducing carbs and eating 'fat to satiety' is a simple way to move away from the fat and carb danger zone.
- Once your progress stalls, it's then time to reduce dietary fat. If you want to increase <u>satiety</u> further, manage your appetite and continue to burn body fat.
- 'Eat fat to burn fat' is poor advice that rarely leads to more optimal body composition in the long term.

Keto Lie #4: Protein Should Be Avoided Due to Gluconeogenesis.

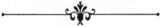

Perhaps the biggest differentiator between keto and other successful versions of a lower-carb diet like Atkins, Paleo, Bernstein, Banting, and Carnivore is the misguided fear that 'excess protein' keeps ketones low and insulin high through the process of gluconeogenesis.

Ever since the keto gurus discovered that <u>protein could convert to glucose via gluconeogenesis</u> and, therefore, lower blood ketones, many low-carb and keto groups have been confused about and afraid of protein. Many keto gurus recommend doing whatever you can to minimise protein and replace those calories with fat to maximise ketosis, believing that protein would effectively turn into chocolate cake in your blood.

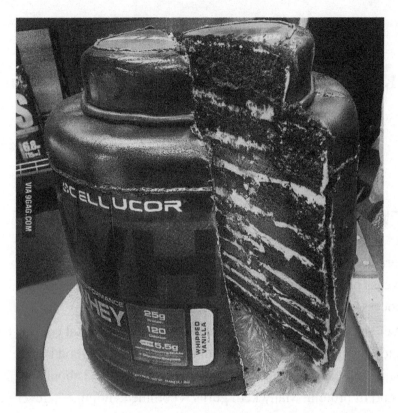

Sadly, many of these people can't work out why their weight loss has stalled with the belief that protein is bad and fat is good, despite 'doing everything right'.

How Do We Measure Protein Intake?

Before we get into recommended protein quantities, we should touch on how protein intake is measured. A lot of confusion comes from mixing up the different units used to measure protein. However, the reality is that people are often talking about almost the same protein intake in practice.

The table below shows some examples of different protein recommendations. People talk about protein in terms of body weight, lean body mass (LBM), ideal body weight, or percentages. Some people talk about protein per kilogram, while others talk about it per pound.

	Metric	Pros	Cons
Total body weight	g/kg BW g/lb BW	Easy to measure because most people don't measure their body fat.	Doesn't consider body fat that is less metabolically active.
Lean body mass (LBM)	g/kg LBM g/lb LBM	More accurate because it accounts for active lean tissue.	Requires some understanding of body fat levels.
Ideal body weight/Reference body weight	g/kg IBW g/lb IBW	Doesn't require the measurement of body fat.	Difficult to agree ideal body weight.
Percentage of calories	%	Simple	Doesn't account for whether you are in an energy surplus or deficit.

Our preference is to use protein per unit of lean body mass (i.e., g/kg or g/lb LBM) because it's your muscles and organs that are metabolically active. On the contrary, your body fat is, for the most part, just your fuel tank that comes along for the ride.

You can use a DEXA scan bioimpedance scale or comparison pictures (like the ones below) to estimate your level of body fat (% BF). DEXA scans are expensive but accurate, whereas bioimpedance scales and comparison pictures are easy to do at home to compare your progress.

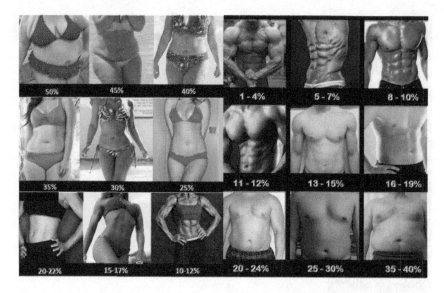

If you're interested, you could calculate your LBM using the following formula:

lean body mass (LBM) = bodyweight x (100% – %BF) / 100%.

Calculating your body fat levels or protein intake with a high degree of accuracy is unnecessary for most people, given that their protein target should generally be treated as a minimum.

To quickly calculate your target protein intake, you can use the simple macro calculator here.

What Is the Absolute Minimum Protein Intake Required?

According to Cahill's starvation studies, we burn about 0.4 g/kg LBM per day of protein via gluconeogenesis during prolonged starvation.

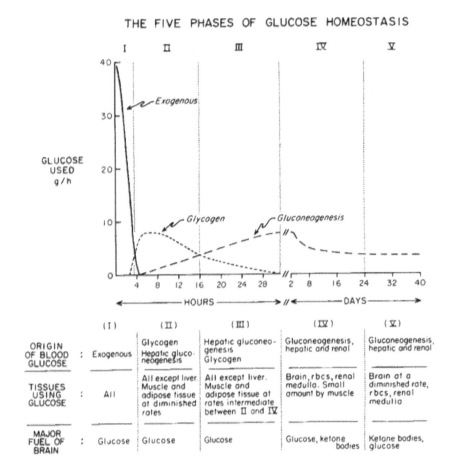

THE FIVE PHASES OF GLUCOSE HOMEOSTASIS

	(I)	(II)	(III)	(IV)	(V)
ORIGIN OF BLOOD GLUCOSE :	Exogenous	Glycogen Hepatic gluco-neogenesis	Hepatic gluconeo-genesis Glycogen	Gluconeogenesis, hepatic and renal	Gluconeogenesis, hepatic and renal
TISSUES USING GLUCOSE :	All	All except liver. Muscle and adipose tissue at diminished rates	All except liver. Muscle and adipose tissue at rates intermediate between II and IV	Brain, rbcs, renal medulla. Small amount by muscle	Brain at a diminished rate, rbcs, renal medulla
MAJOR FUEL OF BRAIN :	Glucose	Glucose	Glucose	Glucose, ketone bodies	Ketone bodies, glucose

After we burn through the food in our stomach and the glycogen stores in our liver and muscles, the body will turn to its internal protein stores from muscles, organs, and, to a lesser extent, the glycerol backbone of fatty acids to obtain glucose via gluconeogenesis.

The figure below shows how we use less protein for energy the longer we go without food (from *Quantitative Physiology of Human Starvation: Adaptations of Energy Expenditure, Macronutrient Metabolism and Body Composition*). After a couple of days without food, fat supplies and ketosis kick in to supply the energy deficit.

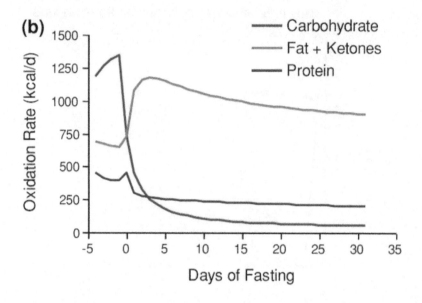

(b)

In the first few days, you will be using around 400 calories from protein or about 100 grams of protein per day. Over the long term, this decreases to 250 calories worth or roughly 60 grams of protein per day.

While protein requirements reduce during extended fasting, this amount of protein you are pulling from your muscles and organs is still significant. Therefore, if you fast for a couple of days every week, you will need to make up for that protein across the week to prevent a long-term loss of lean muscle.

When you refeed, your body will seek out foods to replenish the energy and nutrients it has lost. So, if you do not prioritise protein when you refeed, you will consume more energy to get the protein that your body requires as your body drives you to eat more. But the unfortunate reality is that when we get ravenous after not eating for a long time, we tend to gravitate to energy-dense, lower protein foods, so we struggle to make up for our protein deficit after fasting.

This is why so many people lose and regain the same weight when they attempt extended fasting without paying attention to food quality when they refeed. Regardless of how long you choose to fast, nutrient-focused refeeding (especially protein!) is critical.

Over the short term, gluconeogenesis and autophagy are not necessarily bad. Your body increases autophagy (self-eating) to use the old, sick, and redundant body parts as fuel. After a fast, the body is primed, highly insulin sensitive, and ready to build new muscle.

The reality is that most people see their lean mass drop during any form of energy restriction. This includes extended fasting. It's ideal if you can keep an eye on your changes in lean mass over time.

While no method of measuring body fat is entirely accurate, tracking your change against your baseline with tools like bioimpedance scales that you can use at home every day will give you an understanding of whether you should increase your protein intake if you find you are losing muscle rather than fat.

The Minimum Amount of Protein to Prevent Diseases of Deficiency

The Daily Recommended Intake (DRI) for protein is 0.84 g/kg of body weight (BW), while the Estimated Average Requirement (EAR) is 0.68 g/kg BW. However, it's critical to keep in mind that the DRI is a recommended *minimum* amount needed per day to prevent diseases of protein deficiency.

Recent studies have indicated that higher quantities of protein may be necessary, especially in older people. They may require up to 1.2 to 2.0 g/kg of BW of protein per day to optimise physical function.

According to Raubenheimer and Simpson older people tend to require more dietary protein because they are more likely to be insulin resistant. Thus, they are more likely to have excessive levels of gluconeogenesis (*Obesity: the protein leverage hypothesis*) causing the protein they eat to be transformed and 'lost' as glucose in the bloodstream.

On another note, your body will make the glucose it needs from the protein you eat if you are only consuming minimal amounts of carbs. Hence, you may require extra protein to supply your body with the glucose it needs. If you don't prioritise adequate dietary protein, your appetite will increase to ensure you get enough protein, even if you have to consume more energy than you require.

Rather than avoiding protein, it's better to target a higher protein *percentage* (protein %) if your goal is to lower your insulin, reduce body fat, and improve your insulin sensitivity. A diet with a higher protein percentage also improves satiety. In time, it can lead to fat loss, lowered blood sugar, and normalised insulin levels.

Minimum Protein to Grow Muscle

You'll need more protein for growth and repair if you're active. If you're sedentary, you'll need less. Most of the time, our appetite sorts this out for us, and we may crave more protein if we are doing a lot of resistance training. If you're active, your appetite for protein will likely increase to ensure you get enough of it to prevent muscle loss.

As shown in the figure below from the study, *Effects of Exercise on Dietary Protein Requirements (Lemon, 1999)*:

- a strength athlete requires at least 1.8 g/kg body weight to maximise muscle protein synthesis.
- an endurance athlete should consume at least 1.4 g/kg body weight; and
- someone who is sedentary needs at least 0.9 g/kg body weight.

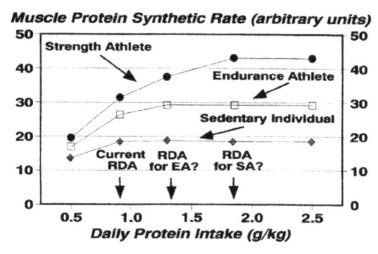

Figure 13 — Proposed effects of increasing dietary protein on muscle protein synthetic rate in sedentary individuals versus endurance and strength athletes. The synthetic rate plateaus in sedentary individuals around the RDA (0.8 g · kg⁻¹ · day⁻¹) and does not increase further with greater protein intakes. In strength athletes the protein synthetic rate plateaus at much greater intakes (perhaps as high as 1.7 g · kg⁻¹ · day⁻¹), indicating that the RDA for this group should be at or near this intake (approximately two times the current RDA). Endurance athletes likely fall somewhere in between the other two groups. Based on data from References 57 and 76.

Note: These values should be seen as <u>minimums</u> during weight maintenance. More protein may increase satiety, improve nutrient density, and decrease the loss of lean mass when losing fat.

How Much Protein Do You Need to Prevent Muscle Loss?

If you are active or incorporating resistance training, you will have a greater protein requirement in an energy deficit for fat loss. Using data from a review paper by Stuart Phillips, lean muscle mass is best preserved when we have at least 2.6 g/kg total body weight with an aggressive deficit (e.g., 35%). On the contrary, a lower protein intake of 1.5 g/kg body weight seems adequate where we have a less aggressive deficit.

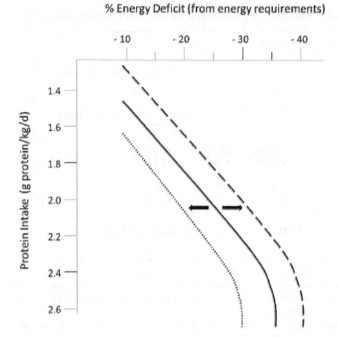

Figure 3: Hypothetical illustration of protein requirements to spare lean mass increasing with greater energy deficits. A rightward shift of the curve (dashed line) indicates lower protein requirements. Similarly, a leftward shift of the curve (dotted line), indicates greater protein requirements. The plateau in the lines demonstrates that with decreasing energy intake, increased protein intake becomes less effective to spare lean mass.

Does Protein Raise Blood Sugars?

Many people are concerned that protein will raise their blood sugars. However, foods with more protein are often lower in carbohydrates, which tend to drive up blood sugars the most. This is shown in the chart below from our analysis of the Food Insulin Index data.

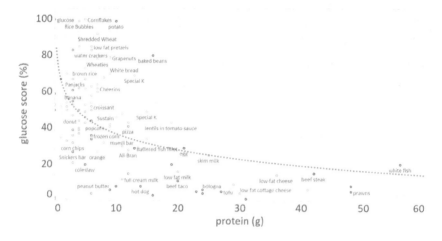

Foods relatively higher in protein also tend to displace carbohydrates in the diet. Our analysis of the Food Insulin Index data also shows that protein does not influence blood sugars post-meal (see *What affects your blood sugar and insulin (other than carbs?*).

While protein *can* be converted to glucose, this does not occur immediately. When you eat protein, your pancreas secretes glucagon. Glucagon pushes liver glycogen into your bloodstream as glucose. The glycogen response is balanced by insulin, and blood sugar thus remains stable for most people.

Many metabolically healthy people find their blood sugars *decrease* after a high-protein, low-carb meal because of the insulin response they get from protein. This is especially true after a high-protein morning meal when their body is primed to store energy after an overnight fast.

Conversely, people who are insulin resistant may find the insulin they release in response to protein does not act as effectively to balance the glucagon. As a result, they may see their blood sugars rise.

Some people see this rise in blood glucose as a reason to avoid protein. Because a significant amount of their dietary protein is being used to supply the glucose they need, they must instead shift their focus to getting *enough* protein to ensure enough amino acids are available for muscle protein synthesis and other critical bodily functions. This excess gluconeogenesis can cause their appetite to ramp up to ensure they get the protein they need.

If you see your blood sugars rise significantly after a low-carb, high-protein meal, you likely have a significant amount of insulin resistance because you are above your Personal Fat Threshold. Rather than avoiding protein and prioritising fat in a misguided effort to improve your insulin resistance, you actually need to do the opposite!

Insulin Dosing for Dietary Protein

Type-1 Diabetics following a low-carb diet know that they require extra insulin for dietary protein as well as carbohydrates.

Because insulin works to build and repair your muscles and keep your stored energy locked away while eating, you will need a little extra insulin several hours after consuming a high-protein meal.

Over the first three hours, protein requires about half as much insulin as carbohydrates. However, as we will learn later, the fact that protein requires bolus insulin, or the insulin associated with the food we eat, should not be of concern.

Protein promotes satiety, which will allow your stored body fat to be used. Protein will also reduce your basal insulin requirements and total insulin demand throughout the day.

Adjusting Diabetes Medications

Injected insulin helps manage the symptoms of Type-2 Diabetes, like elevated blood sugars, but it does little to reverse the underlying cause of energy toxicity. In addition, because insulin is the hormone that tells our liver to hold back energy in storage, exogenous insulin also tends to make it harder to lose unwanted body fat.

Injected insulin forces your body to hold fat in storage, resulting in hunger and resultant weight gain. As you lose weight, you will see your need for both injected basal and bolus insulin reduce as you lose excess body fat and improve your insulin sensitivity.

If you are taking any diabetes-related medications like injected insulin, you should pay particular attention to your blood sugars and work with your healthcare team to adjust your medications to ensure that your blood sugars don't go lower than 4.0 mmol/L (72 mg/dL). You will not only feel unwell below this level, but you will likely want to eat anything, and everything until your blood sugar returns to normal.

Establishing a predictable routine is crucial if you are taking diabetes medications. If you radically change your eating pattern by suddenly skipping a whole day of eating or engaging in multi-day fasts, your insulin needs will plummet, and you will risk low blood sugar or hypoglycemia.

Why Protein Percentage Is More Useful

Optimising Nutrition advisor Dr Ted Naiman has recently been advocating for more intelligent consideration of the Protein:Energy Ratio (P: E). This ratio is based on the Protein Leverage Hypothesis, which demonstrates that all living organisms, including humans, eat until they get the protein they need.

Optimising the macronutrient composition of your diet for greater satiety is the key to managing your food intake with less willpower and self-imposed deprivation.

- The key to increasing satiety and eating less is to *increase* your protein PERCENTAGE (protein %), or your number of total calories from protein.
- Conversely, the way to eat more to grow and fuel high activity levels is to *decrease* your protein percentage by increasing your intake of energy from fat and carbs.

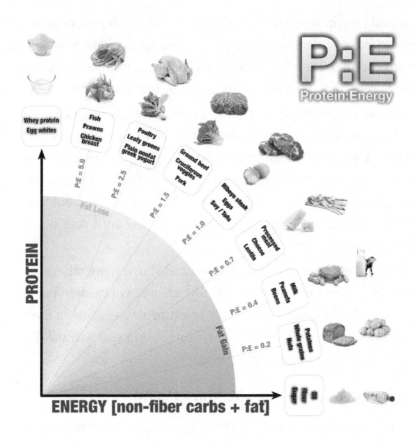

Our analysis of half a million days of data from MyFitnessPal users and 125,761 days of macronutrient and micronutrient data from 34,519 people who have used Nutrient Optimiser further supports the Protein Leverage Hypothesis.

Of all the quantifiable factors, *protein percentage* of your diet has the most significant impact on satiety of all the macronutrients and essential micronutrients. And yes, we have tested them all!

The chart below shows the relationship between protein % and calorie intake from our Optimiser data, showing that as we move from a low protein % to a high protein %, we tend to consume 55% fewer calories!

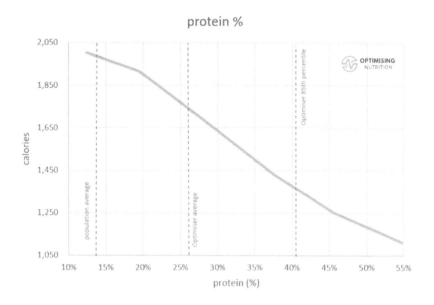

protein %

Managing your appetite and spontaneously eating less is not necessarily about eating more protein. Instead, you can incrementally dial up the *percentage* of protein in your diet by reducing your intake of fat and carbs while prioritising protein.

The chart below shows the relationship between protein %, protein (in grams), and total calorie intake. Moving from 15% to 50% protein aligns with:

- a total reduction of 800 calories,
- an increase in protein of 75 g (or 300 calories), and
- a reduction of 1100 calories from fat and carbs.

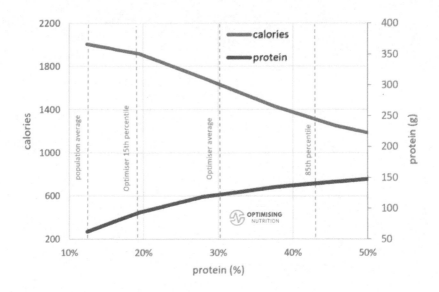

By contrast, many low-carb or keto communities advocate the exact opposite to break a fat loss stall, recommending that you avoid protein because of its short-term impact on insulin and eat more fat to increase ketones. Meanwhile, many in the low-fat or plant-based communities also recommend actively avoiding protein for various reasons.

Although we live in a postmodern world where everyone is entitled to their own opinion that may be overly skewed from their own personal social media feed, science and human metabolism are the same regardless of our beliefs.

Our data analysis of 125,761 days of macronutrient and micronutrient data from 34,519 people who have used Nutrient Optimiser also shows that our overall calorie intake decreases as our *percentage* of protein increases. It is challenging to overconsume foods with a higher percentage of protein. Sadly, the average population's 13-15% protein intake aligns with the *lowest satiety* response.

However, it's not sustainable to jump from 10 to 50% of your total calories from protein overnight. Instead, slowly increasing your protein percentage by dialling back readily accessible energy from fat and carbohydrates is a more sustainable way to lose fat from your body.

Analysis of our data from <u>Nutrient Optimiser</u> users shows that most people prioritising <u>nutrient density</u> consume around 1.8 g/kg LBM protein. In our <u>Macros Masterclass,</u> we tend to see the best satiety response and the quickest weight loss when people consume this amount of protein as a minimum and dial back their fat and carb intakes progressively.

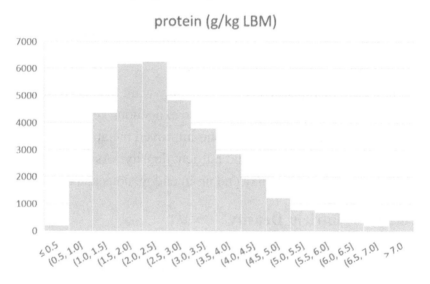

protein (g/kg LBM)

Prioritising adequate dietary protein ensures you don't lose precious, metabolically active muscle and other crucial lean mass like your vital organs. Reducing dietary carbs helps decrease blood sugar variability, whereas reducing dietary fat helps promote body fat loss and leads to lower blood sugars over the long term.

Will Too Much Protein 'Kick Me Out of Ketosis'?

Studies tend to be mixed on whether higher levels of protein decrease ketones. However, many people anecdotally report that their ketones do decrease with higher levels of dietary protein.

This makes logical sense, given that protein provides oxaloacetate. Oxaloacetate enables fat to be burned in the citric acid cycle rather than through ketosis, which is a less efficient process. However, you must consider your goals to understand whether or not you need to be concerned about decreased ketones.

- Do you want to achieve *exogenous ketosis*, or measurable amounts of ketones from added dietary fat so that you can achieve therapeutic levels of ketones for the management of epilepsy, Alzheimer's or dementia.

- are you aiming for *endogenous ketosis*, where the body produces ketones for fat loss, improved metabolic health, or diabetes management?

If you require therapeutic ketosis, you may want to keep your protein low and add dietary fat to force exogenous ketosis. However, if your goal is fat loss and improved metabolic health, you should prioritise satiety and nutrient density. As a side effect of burning body fat, you may end up in endogenous ketosis.

Protein vs Nutrient Density

Foods with a higher percentage of protein tend to be more nutritious. For whatever reason, the fear of protein has led people to eat more from low satiety.

People negating protein get fewer critical nutrients (like amino acids) from their food and crave more food to compensate. This perpetuates an unhealthy eating cycle that perpetuates a paradox of overeating (energy) while still suffering from nutrient deficiency. As shown in the chart below, up to about 50%, a higher protein percentage correlates with a greater nutrient density.

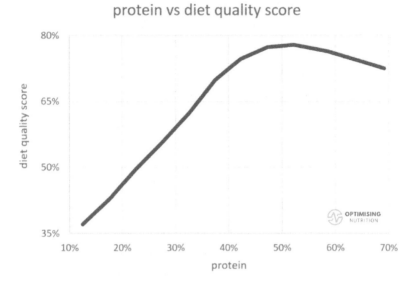

protein vs diet quality score

If you design your diet to achieve high ketone levels as the primary goal, you are also prone to nutrient deficiencies and inherent cravings that result from your body trying to get the protein and nutrients it requires.

What About Protein Powders?

Protein powders can provide bioavailable protein that enables you to top your intake up if you are struggling to get enough. This is a great way for active people to get enough energy and protein to support their activity levels or grow bigger and stronger.

Jose Antonio has led numerous studies where they have tried to overfeed active people with up to 4.4 g protein/kg/day, or five times the recommended daily protein allowance.

The first observation in these studies was that people struggle to eat that much protein, even from processed powders. The second observation was that the participants did not gain weight or body fat despite consuming more calories. This is because the body struggles to convert dietary protein to body fat.

The downside is that protein powders and all the food products that contain them won't provide you with the same array of nutrients as whole foods. While they provide heaps of amino acids per calorie, they don't provide a high level of vitamins and minerals as their whole food counterparts.

Perhaps most importantly, powders don't provide the same satiety as whole food protein sources. Whey protein is a 'waste' that is produced during the cheese-making process. Because it is already highly processed, your body doesn't need to do much work to convert it to usable energy. Thus, dietary-induced thermogenesis is much lower for protein powders than minimally processed forms of protein found in whole foods.

As always, do whatever you can to prioritise nutrient-dense whole foods and use supplementary protein powders as a last resort.

Is Too Much Protein Bad for my Kidneys?

One of the primary functions of your kidneys is to filter your blood. The *estimated* glomerular filtration rate (eGFR) is a standard test that indicates how well your kidneys are working. The eGFR is based on the amount of creatine—the substance produced from the breakdown of protein found in your muscles—in your bloodstream.

Some people become concerned when they see high eGFR levels and think the protein they're eating is causing kidney dysfunction. However, it shouldn't be surprising that people eating more protein often carry more muscle than average.

People supplementing with creatine may also see higher creatinine in their bloodstream. Creatine is found in meat and fish, and it is one of the most well-researched and beneficial supplements for strength, cognitive performance, and even allergies.

We don't tend to see active bodybuilders getting kidney failure *because of* their high-protein diets. Instead, it is often the other way around: high-protein diets are often a problem if the kidneys have a pre-existing condition.

If you have late-stage kidney failure and are on dialysis, it's worth talking to your nephrologist about how much protein they think you should be consuming. But if you don't already have a nephrologist, then it's unlikely that 'too much protein' will be a concern for your kidneys.

Most people on kidney dialysis have pre-existing elevated blood sugar and blood pressure. According to Dr Ted Naiman, people consuming more protein tend to have larger, higher functioning kidneys. Eating more protein is akin to beneficial 'resistance training' for your kidneys. Similar to how you want to avoid your muscles weakening from disuse, you don't want your kidneys to atrophy with age.

In a 2018 meta-analysis titled *Changes in Kidney Function Do Not Differ between Healthy Adults Consuming Higher- Compared with Lower- or Normal-Protein Diets: A Systematic Review and Meta-Analysis* by Professor Stuart Phillips, it was found that increased protein intakes do not adversely influence kidney function in healthy adults.

What About 'Rabbit Starvation'?

'Rabbit starvation' is a term used to describe what happens to lean and active people when they prioritise lean protein foods and minimise their intake of fat and carbohydrates.

The term originated from active pioneers and explorers who had to live on available game meat, which was often lean. While rabbits are plentiful, they contain meagre amounts of fat.

Therefore, people living on rabbits alone find it difficult to consume enough energy to sustain even low body fat levels. But for most of us with plenty of body fat to burn, this is not an issue! Once we get adequate protein, our appetite for high-protein foods shuts down, and we search for easily-accessible energy from fat and carbs.

If you are getting super lean and only have high-protein foods available to eat, 'rabbit starvation' may be an issue for you. But as long as you have a significant amount of body fat to burn, 'rabbit starvation' is not something to be concerned about.

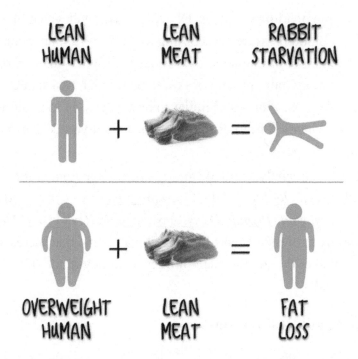

Summary

If your only goal is elevated blood ketones, keeping your protein intake low may help. However, prioritising a higher *percentage* of protein in your diet is a better approach regardless of ketone levels if your goal is fat loss, improved metabolic health, or diabetes reversal.

Keto Lie #5: Fat is a 'Free Food' Because it Doesn't Elicit an Insulin Response.

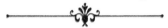

This is one of the cornerstone beliefs of many low-carb and keto diet subscribers.

Many theorise that because carbohydrates raise insulin, the most and insulin is related to fat storage, eating more carbohydrates will lead to greater body fat storage.

Thus, dietary fat should be the primary energy source because it doesn't impact blood sugar or insulin levels and is effectively a 'free food'.

Will More Insulin Make You Fat?

Essentially, the <u>Carbohydrate-Insulin Hypothesis</u> says:

eat more carbohydrates -> make more insulin -> get fatter

Dr <u>David Ludwig</u> states that '<u>insulin is like Miracle-Gro for your fat cells</u>'. Dr Jason Fung says, '<u>I can make you fat. I can make anybody fat. I just need to give you enough insulin</u>'.

This theory is partially correct. If someone injects excessive amounts of exogenous insulin, their liver will hold their stored energy back, and the energy in their bloodstream will decrease. They will soon become *extremely* hungry, compelling them to eat more. As a result, they will eat an excessive amount of food and gain fat.

However, this 'fun fact' is utterly irrelevant for the 98.5% of the population with a working pancreas.

Unless you are injecting insulin to manage Type-1 Diabetes or advanced Type-2 Diabetes, this is entirely irrelevant! It would be illegal for someone to jab you with a needle and inject you with insulin throughout the day. They would be deemed a dangerous public nuisance and locked up.

On another note, your body is super-efficient. It does not produce more of anything than it needs. When consuming food, your pancreas will not release more insulin than it requires to keep your stowed energy in storage.

As shown in the chart below, total insulin demand across the day is positively correlated with your body mass index (BMI)underline. While correlation does not necessarily mean causation, it appears that your insulin requirement throughout the day is driven by the amount of stored energy your body is holding.

Insulin and Body Mass Index

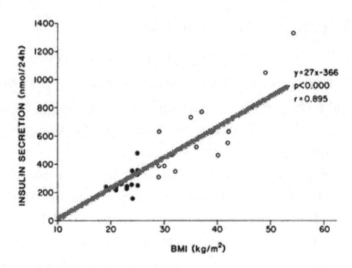

For a more detailed discussion of this topic, see underline What Does Insulin Do in Your Body?underline

Basal vs Bolus Insulin

People with Type-1 Diabetes know they must use basal insulin to keep their blood sugars stable when they don't eat and bolus insulin to compensate for their food and meals.

For people on a standard high-carb diet, basal insulin makes up around 50% of their total daily insulin. The rest is injected to manage their meals. However, for someone following a low-carb or keto diet, basal insulin can make up as much as 90% of their total daily insulin requirements.

Unless you let your blood sugars run high by switching off your insulin pump or choosing not to take your injections, the only way to reduce the insulin produced by your pancreas is to focus on eating high-satiety foods. This will allow you to consume less energy without having to exert unsustainable levels of willpower.

We Don't Really Understand the Long-Term Insulin Response to Food

It is true that your pancreas produces more insulin acutely in response to carbohydrates, followed by protein and then fat. *Note: Fructose and fibre tend to have lower insulin demand relative to carbohydrates.*

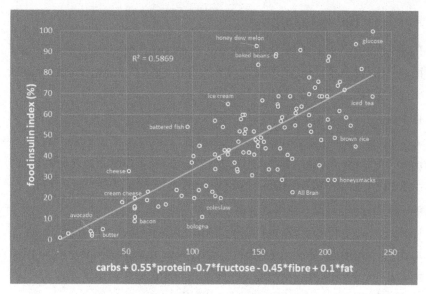

For more detail, see <u>What affects your blood sugar and insulin (other than carbs)?</u> for more details.

The data from <u>Food Insulin Index</u> testing suggests that fat has about 10% of the insulin response that carbs do. However, it's critical to keep in mind these insulin tests only look at the first two hours after eating.

We know *very little* about the long-term insulin response to the foods we eat after those two hours, but it appears that fat elicits a significant insulin response in the fullness of time.

To illustrate, the chart below shows how different macronutrient ratios elicit different blood sugar responses by comparing a 75% carbohydrate plant-based low-fat (PBLF) diet (green line) vs a 75% fat animal-based low-carb (ABLC) diet (red line). Blood glucose rises quickly in response to low-fat foods, whereas it increases slowly from low-carb foods. However, blood sugars for both extremes are still elevated above the baseline after two hours.

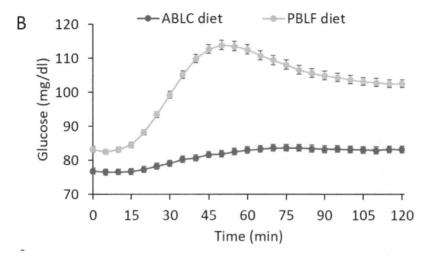

Data from: A plant-based, low-fat diet decreases ad libitum energy intake compared to an animal-based, ketogenic diet: An inpatient randomised controlled trial

Blood sugars and insulin rise and fall more quickly in response to a high-carb meal than to a high-fat meal. While it's likely that less insulin is produced in response to fat as opposed to carbohydrates, the insulin response to fat is still significant if we're considering things calorie-for-calorie and in the fullness of time.

After watching Moni's closed-loop pump system for years, I know anecdotally that a large steak will require continual insulin for *up to 10 hours* as it's digested and metabolised. But if she ever happens to eat something that combines carbs and fat, her insulin requirements will be elevated for more than a day, and she will need more insulin to keep her blood sugars suppressed.

A lot is going on beyond the two hours we have measurements for. Hence, we can't assume that there is a negligible insulin response to high-fat foods.

Oxidative Priority

A little-known fact when it comes to nutrition and metabolism is that the order your body burns the various fuels in your body and the amount of insulin released is proportional to the capacity your body has to store each of them.

This is known as <u>oxidative priority or oxidative hierarchy</u>. The table below shows the relative priority that alcohol, ketones, glucose, and fat are used in your body.

	Alcohol	Ketones	Excess protein	Glucose	Fatty acids	Body fat
Priority	1	2	3	4	5	6
Use	Energy	Energy	Energy and excretion	Energy	Energy	Storage
Capacity (calories)	20	20	-	1200 – 2000	150	40,000 – 500,000
Thermic effect	15%	3%	20 – 35%	5 – 15%	3 – 15%	3 – 15%

Adapted from: *Oxidative Priority, Meal Frequency, and the Energy Economy of Food and Activity: Implications for Longevity, Obesity, and Cardiometabolic Disease* by Cronise et al., 2017.

We have *minimal* capacity to store alcohol, ketones, and any protein in excess of what you require for muscle synthesis and other critical bodily functions. Your body raises insulin to abruptly shut off the release of stored energy until it utilises these fuels.

Your body has *some* capacity to store glucose, but not a lot. Thus, we see an aggressive insulin response to carbohydrates. However, your body is more than happy to hold fat in your adipose tissue (i.e., on your butt, tummy, or muffin top), which is why the insulin response for fat is less acute.

Because fat is less volatile and has a lower <u>thermic effect</u> relative to other fuels, it is much easier to store. While protein and carbs are difficult to convert to fat for storage, it's super easier for the body to store dietary fat as body fat. Thus, any fat that's left over once you've burned through any alcohol, carbs, or excess protein is easily stored as body fat.

The chart below shows a figure that we use in <u>Data-Driven Fasting</u> to explain the interconnected fuel tanks in our bodies. Most of us have our blood glucose and liver glycogen tanks filled to the brim. Your pancreas is working overtime to keep insulin elevated to hold back the fat in storage while burning off the more volatile glucose in your blood.

The SECRET to fat loss

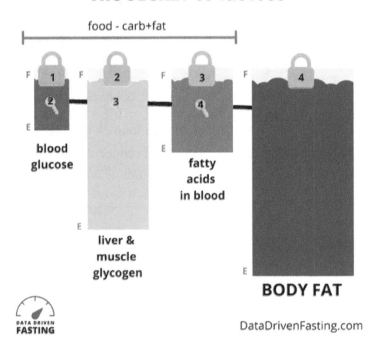

The insulin response to carbohydrates is acute simply because you don't have much room to store glucose in your body. Conversely, the body has a smaller and slower response to fat simply because it has plenty of capacity to store it in large quantities.

However, once we drain our glucose, by waiting a little longer between meals, your body lowers insulin to allow the stored glycogen in your liver to be released into the bloodstream.

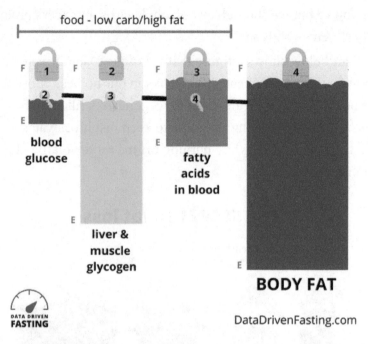

Once your liver glycogen is depleted, so long as you are not overdoing the dietary fat, your body will reduce insulin further to allow your stored body fat to be used, which is what most of us are chasing in the long run.

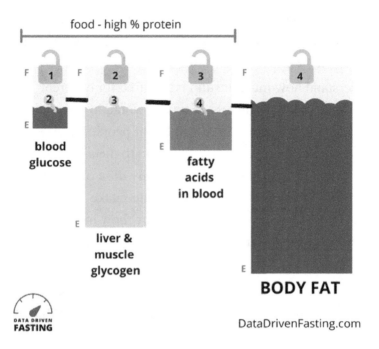

food - high % protein

blood glucose

liver & muscle glycogen

fatty acids in blood

BODY FAT

DataDrivenFasting.com

For more details on this concept, see *Oxidative Priority: The Key to Unlocking Your Body Fat Stores*.

You Can't Turn Off Your Insulin!

Some people with Type-1 Diabetes partake in a dangerous practice called diabulimia which involves intentionally underdosing their insulin so blood sugars run high, and they can lose weight.

Their stored energy rapidly flows into their bloodstream, leading to dangerously high blood sugars, ketones, and free fatty acids in the blood. The potentially life-threatening state known as Diabetic Ketoacidosis and horrific levels of muscle wastage can also result.

When my wife Monica was first diagnosed with Type-1 Diabetes, she was losing 0.5 kg per day! She would have wasted away and died in just a few days without exogenous insulin.

I'm explaining this horrific process because this is what people who believe in the Carbohydrate-Insulin Hypothesis think will happen to them when they reduce dietary carbohydrates. But this is not the case, and they don't understand what they are hoping for. Uncontrolled Type-1 Diabetes is a truly terrible disease, and you can't bring it upon yourself by simply avoiding carbs and protein!

To understand how much insulin is required for different macronutrients in the fullness of time, I would love to see an experiment done where a large number of people with Type-1 Diabetes following both high- and low-carb diets track their food meticulously and correlate their total daily dose of insulin with their calorie, protein, fat and carbohydrate intake. Until we have the results of such a study, we won't know how much insulin is precisely required throughout the day for different macronutrients. What we do know is that:

- the limited insulin data that we have only considered the first two hours after eating. Thus, the full insulin demand of our food is still very poorly understood, especially for fat which has a slower and longer insulin response after eating.
- because your body must first burn off carbs and excess protein, more insulin is released to stop the breakdown of stored body fat while you use up the fuels it can't store much of. Meanwhile, it is easy to store fat, and you have a lot of room to store it. Hence, the insulin response after eating it is much lower.
- most of the insulin produced by your pancreas is required to hold your fat in storage. Therefore, the best way to reduce insulin is to find a way of eating that allows you to eat less without excessive self-restraint.

How to Reduce Your Insulin Levels Across the Day

While we don't have data showing the long-term responses to different macronutrients, I do have Monica's total daily insulin dosage data from the past ten years.

This chart shows how her insulin requirements have changed as we've progressed from a standard higher-carb diet to a low-carb diet to a low insulin load. However, her lowest insulin requirements were when she participated in our Macros Masterclass in January 2019.

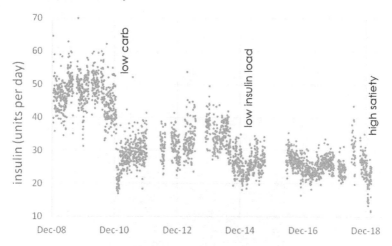

The chart below shows Monica's insulin dose in the period leading up to and during the first Macros Masterclass that we did together. As you can see, her daily insulin demand dropped from the high twenties to the teens.

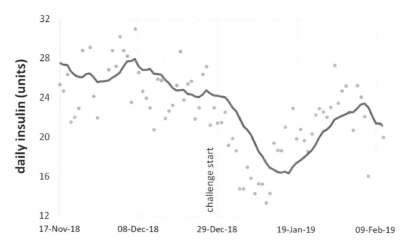

To be clear, Type-1 Diabetes cannot be cured or reversed. Monica's pancreas still produces no insulin. However, the insulin she requires was vastly reduced by optimising her food choices and reducing her body fat levels.

During the Masterclass, Monica lost 7.5 kg (16.5 lbs) or 10.7% of her body weight during the six-week challenge. These photos show us both before and after those six weeks.

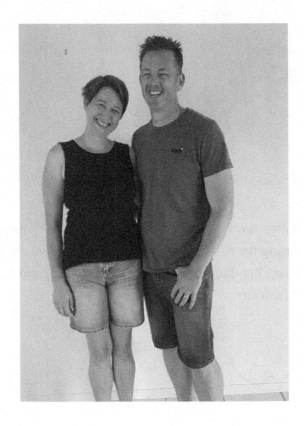

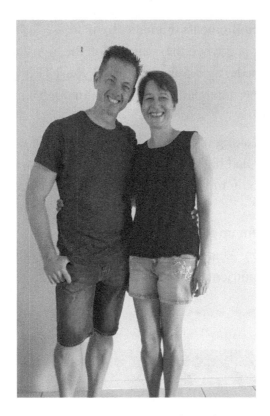

The main difference from Monica's previous diet was a reduced intake of nuts, cheese, and cream which are helpful foods to stabilise blood sugars. However, they are not ideal for fat loss or reducing insulin throughout the day.

Although high-fat foods elicit a slower and more stable insulin response, they still affect insulin requirements across the whole day. While low-carb foods like nuts, cheese, and cream are excellent foods for people managing diabetes to obtain adequate energy and maintain stable blood sugars, they also appear to trigger a long-term insulin response and prevent blood sugar levels from dropping below the threshold that fat burning starts.

Reducing those foods improves satiety, reduces overall energy intake, which lowers insulin across the day and allows body fat to be used.

Anecdotally, others with Type-1 Diabetes have shared that their daily insulin requirements dramatically increased, and their insulin sensitivity dropped when they jumped on the high-fat keto trend. Allison Herschede, a co-founder of the <u>Type-1 Grit Facebook Group</u>, found her total daily dose of insulin *doubled* on a 90% fat keto style diet.

Allison said, 'Taking my insulin was like injecting water. I realised the only time I had high ketone levels was when I was insulin resistant. The only time I ever had high ketones was when I was eating 90% fat'.

Her HbA1c went up to 8% during her high-fat keto experimentation. Thankfully, it has now returned to 4.8% after following our nutrient-dense, high-satiety meals.

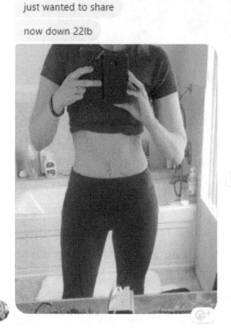

Focusing on <u>nutrient-dense</u>, high-<u>satiety</u> foods tends to reduce overall insulin requirements across the day and not just immediately after meals.

By focusing on <u>nutrient density</u>, you are also able to get the nutrients you need with fewer calories and improve satiety!

What is Really Happening?

Rather than:

> *eating more carbohydrates -> making more insulin -> getting fatter*

driving obesity, it appears to be fuelled by:

> *eating low satiety nutrient-poor foods -> increased cravings and appetite -> increased energy intake -> fat storage -> increased daily insulin*

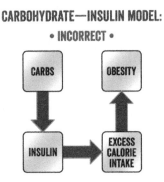 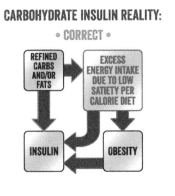

Although it is only *symptom management,* reducing the processed carbs in your diet will help stabilise your blood sugars. However, if you want to lower your insulin requirements, <u>reverse Type-2</u>

<u>Diabetes,</u> and attack energy toxicity—the root cause of most of metabolic diseases—you should prioritise nutrient-dense, high-satiety foods and meals that allow you to reduce your insulin levels throughout the whole day.

The real solution to managing Type-2 Diabetes, blood sugar, insulin levels and avoiding the myriad complications of metabolic syndrome is:

> *consuming high-satiety nutrient-dense foods and meals >
> decreased cravings and appetite -> decreased energy
> intake -> fat loss -> optimised insulin levels*

Keto Lie #6: Food Quality is Not Important. It's all About Reducing Insulin and Avoiding Carbs.

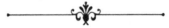

People in Ketoland like to point out 'there is no such thing as an essential carbohydrate'. However, the reality is that many nutrient-dense foods that happen to contain some carbohydrates are also loaded with essential nutrients that are harder to find when carbs are reduced.

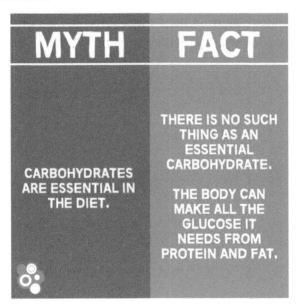

We *do* need some essential fatty acids. However, the actual quantity that you require is tiny, only amounting to 1.6 g of omega-3 and 4.6 g of omega-6 PUFAs or less than 50 calories per day in total.

You only require about 10 g of fat per day to maintain gallbladder function, which equates to less than 90 calories, or 4.5% of your daily energy intake.

You can create a diet of reasonable nutrient density with as little as 10% of the calories coming from fat.

Why Should You Reduce Your Carbs?

Stabilising blood sugars to healthy, non-diabetic levels is a great starting point for your journey towards Nutritional Optimisation. The satiety improvement that comes from stabilising blood sugars to healthy levels is a crucial reason why a keto or low-carb diet works so well for many people, especially when starting from a hyperpalatable, modern, processed diet that mixes refined carbs and processed fats.

- Moving away from the fat and carb danger zone tends to improve satiety and reduce appetite.

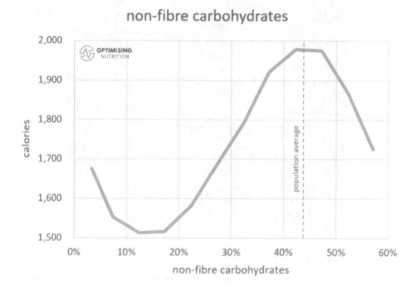

non-fibre carbohydrates

- Foods with less refined carbohydrates tend to contain more bioavailable protein, making us feel fuller with fewer calories (i.e., greater satiety).

- If your blood sugars swing wildly across the day, you will feel compelled to eat again when your blood sugars come crashing down.

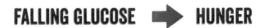

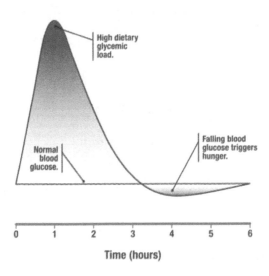

Time (hours)

If you see your blood glucose levels rise by more than 1.6 mmol/L (30 mg/dL) after you eat, you're simply overfilling your glucose fuel tank in your body. So, it's a great idea to reduce the amount of refined carbohydrates in your diet until your blood sugars stabilise to healthy non-diabetic levels.

But beyond worrying about the balance of carbs and fat in your diet, it's ideal to think in terms of a cost-benefit analysis. You simply need to ensure you are getting the nutrients you need without overconsuming energy. We like to call this nutrient density.

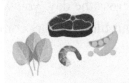

"Your diet doesn't need a name or a belief system, just enough nutrients."

Marty Kendall

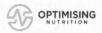

What is Nutrient Density?

Nutrient density is simply the amount of essential nutrients per calorie in a food or meal (i.e., nutrients/calorie).

While calories are not a perfect measure, they are the best litmus we have to compare the nutrients contained in a food, recipe, or a group of foods contains that someone might eat in a day.

Thinking in terms of nutrients per serving or per meal can be helpful if you don't have fat-loss goals. However, nutrients per calorie is highly effective to get enough nutrients for less energy, so you can get on with using body fat for fuel.

Why is Nutrient Density Critical?

Essential micronutrients, or vitamins, minerals, amino acids, and essential fatty acids, are critical to the biochemical processes that power your mitochondria and drive every bodily function to ensure you use energy efficiently. Prioritising foods with a higher nutrient density will ensure you get the vitamins, minerals, amino acids, and fatty acids without having to consume excess energy.

In times gone by, there was no need to worry about nutrient density. Readily available foods contained plenty of the nutrients we needed in the proper ratios. In addition, our highly developed appetite, which works with our other senses like smell, taste, sight/colour, touch/mouthfeel, and hearing/crunch, ensures we get the nutrients and energy we need.

But these days, the essential nutrients in our food have declined because of our reliance on large-scale agricultural practices. Separating animals from plant crops and replacing manure with synthetic fertiliser has also decreased the microbial diversity and nutrient density of the plants we grow and the animals that eat them.

While we all need adequate nutrients, prioritising nutrient density becomes even more critical when trying to lose weight. Even though you're eating fewer calories, you still require enough nutrients.

Simply trying to eat smaller quantities of the nutrient-poor foods that made you fat will leave you with cravings that often lead to increased hunger, appetite, and cravings for the nutrients you need. Unfortunately, before too long, this leads to rebound bingeing and fat gain.

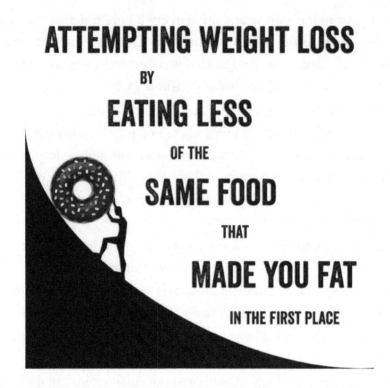

ATTEMPTING WEIGHT LOSS
BY
EATING LESS
OF THE
SAME FOOD
THAT
MADE YOU FAT
IN THE FIRST PLACE

The best-kept weight-loss secret is simple: if you want to lose fat, you must control your appetite by finding a way to get more nutrients per calorie from the food you consume!

How Has Our Food System Changed?

The charts below (created from data from the *USDA Economic Research Service Nutrient Database)* show how the nutrients in our food system have changed over the past century with the increase of chemical fertilisers and reliance on large-scale farming and food manufacturing.

Sodium

Since the mid-1960s, sodium in the US food system has *decreased* significantly. While we are often encouraged to consume less sodium, it's the decrease in sodium over the past 50 years that is most highly correlated with the increase in obesity.

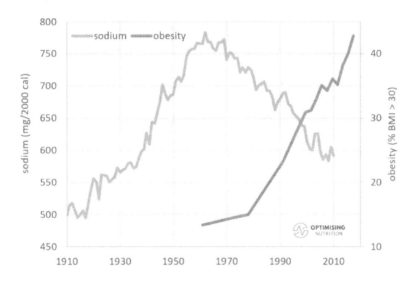

Magnesium

Magnesium has also substantially decreased in parallel with the increase in the use of fertilisers and large-scale agriculture.

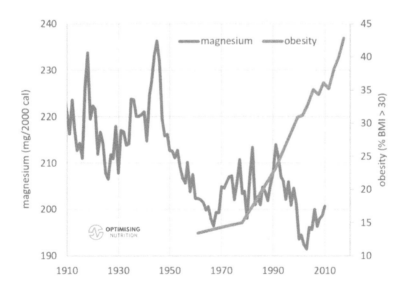

Potassium

As our farmlands have become more depleted, potassium has dropped by around 25%. More recently, we're learning that we're not necessarily overeating sodium, but we're likely consuming too little potassium in pursuit of achieving the optimal potassium: sodium ratio and preventing high blood pressure.

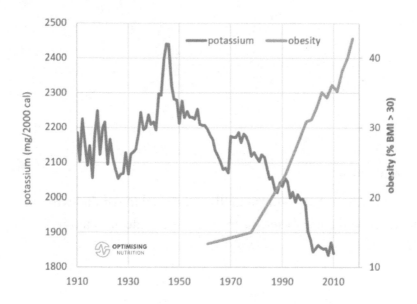

Vitamin A

Vitamin A levels have dropped about 30% since the introduction of the Dietary Goals for Americans in 1977. Rather than simply focusing on the nutrients we require from food; the guidelines encouraged people to avoid their saturated fat and dietary cholesterol.

Ironically, the foods that naturally contain more saturated fat and cholesterol also contain more vitamin A. Avoiding saturated fat in favour of refined grains, sugar, and seed oils has had a devastating impact on our food system's nutrient density.

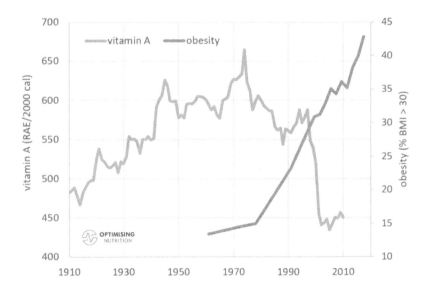

Vitamin B12

Vitamin B12 is an essential nutrient almost exclusively found in animal-based foods that has decreased since the introduction of the 1977 Dietary Guidelines.

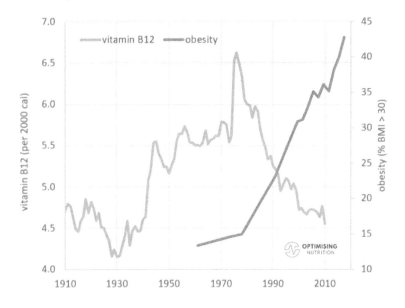

You Need to Eat More to Get the Minimum Nutrient Intake

The table below shows the number of calories you must consume from foods readily available to get the recommended Dietary Reference Intakes for each nutrient listed on a daily basis.

Micronutrient	calories required to meet DRI
Calcium	5400
Potassium	5200
Magnesium	4400

Today, more and more of the foods we consume are precisely engineered formulations of cheap vegetable oils, refined starches, added sugars, flavours, and colours that are designed to look and taste nutritious.

Based on the USDA's latest published data from 2010, 61% of the energy consumed by Americans came from added fats and oils (23%), flours and cereals (23%), and added sugars (15%). Based on the trend over the past half-century, it's likely that this is now even higher. Although these foods are cheap to produce, they are inferior sources of micronutrients.

You'd think nutrition would be primarily about nutrients. But sadly, they are usually an afterthought. Most nutritional advice today focuses on what you should avoid, whether it be too much fat, carbs, protein, saturated fat, sugar, plant-based foods, or animal-based foods.

By focusing on nutrient-dense foods, you ensure you get what you need from the foods you eat. Once you learn to fill your plate with nutrient-dense foods, especially at your first meal of the day, you're much less likely to crave less-than-optimal, nutrient-poor foods that are easy to overeat.

Should I Eat More or Less Fats and Carbs?

The balance of carbs vs fat largely depends on *your* context and goals.

- Carbs are useful for explosive activity as the body uses them to refill your liver and muscles with glycogen if you don't eat a lot of carbohydrates. Although your body can make enough glucose from the protein you eat, it occurs at a slower rate than if carbs were directly ingested.

- Fat is an excellent slow-burning fuel for everyday use. It's great for storage, and typically comes packaged with the protein we eat.

Your choice of fuel must consider *your* goals. To figure out which fuel is best for you, you can ask yourself a few simple questions:

- Do you need to fuel a lot of activity, or are you trying to lose body fat?
- What foods supply you with the nutrients you require while staying within your energy budget?

If you are lean, super active, and your exercise requires short bursts of power, you may crave more carbohydrates to keep your glycogen stores full. While your body can make the glucose it needs from protein, you may benefit from having more dietary carbohydrates if you burn a lot of glucose with explosive activity because this process is rate limited. However, if you are only doing less intense activities, you won't need as many carbohydrates, and fat will steadily supply the energy you need.

If your goal is to lose body fat, your most crucial focus is to ensure you get the nutrients you need without overconsuming energy.

When it comes to carbohydrates, refined grains and starches tend to be nutrient-poor. Hence, they are less-than-optimal food choices. However, although leafy green veggies contain some carbs, they tend to contain many harder-to-find nutrients at the expense of very few calories. Thus, they are a good investment for your limited energy budget.

The fat that comes with protein is typically an excellent source of energy. But you probably should ease up on added fats and oils if you're trying to lose fat from your body.

Once you get leaner and want to continue losing body fat, you may need to look for fewer fatty cuts of meat and fish to ensure you continue burning body fat. Once you have reached your goal weight, you can incorporate more energy from fat or carbs.

In the absence of processed fake foods that contain additives to trick your body into thinking the foods you're eating contain nutrients, your appetite does a pretty good job of seeking out the nutrients you need to thrive without pushing you to overconsume energy.

> **junk food** *noun*
>
> 1. Pre-prepared or packaged food that has low nutritional value
>   —*Oxford English Dictionary*
>
> 2. Food that is not good for your health because it contains high amounts of fat or sugar
>   —*The Merriam-Webster Dictionary*
>
> 3. Food that tastes like something it is not
>   —*Mark Schatzker*

Depending on the circumstances, we often crave different foods at different times to give us the nutrients we need. For example, we may crave:

- more protein after a workout,
- chocolate around 'that time of the month' for women, or
- all sorts of weird and wonderful things if a woman is pregnant to nourish a growing baby.

The Protein Leverage Hypothesis suggests that we keep eating food until we get the protein we require to maintain our muscles. However, it seems that a similar thing occurs with micronutrients to varying extents (as you will see below).

YOU decide WHAT to eat, then YOUR BODY decides HOW MUCH.

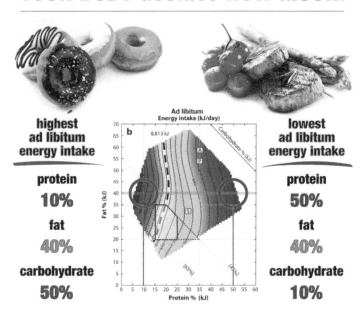

highest ad libitum energy intake		lowest ad libitum energy intake
protein		protein
10%		**50%**
fat		fat
40%		**40%**
carbohydrate		carbohydrate
50%		**10%**

Prioritising nutrient-dense foods will help you reduce your cravings and switch off your appetite once you get enough (but not too much) energy.

In our Micros Masterclass, people who focus on maximising their nutrient density find they are satiated with fewer calories. As a general rule, nutrient-dense foods tend to supply plenty of protein and fibre and contain less fat and carbs. Thus, they are highly satiating and typically hard to overeat.

Satiety vs Nutrient Density

As shown in the nutrient density vs satiety chart below, nutrient-dense foods tend to be more satiating.

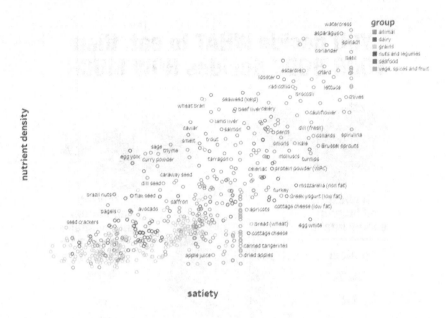

Foods toward the top right of this chart provide plenty of nutrients in exchange for fewer calories and therefore help you manage your appetite with less conscious effort. In contrast, foods like refined grains and fats toward the bottom left tend to increase our appetite, and we must overeat them to obtain adequate nutrients.

If you look closely or check out the interactive Tableau version of the chart here, you will notice that non-starchy vegetables dominate the top right. Non-starchy vegetables are hard to overeat because they are bulky from water and fibre. They are nutrient-dense in terms of nutrients per calorie and highly satiating on a calorie-for-calorie basis. You can think of non-starchy vegetables as nature's vitamin pill.

Although someone following a strict Whole Foods Plant-Based (WFPB) diet may struggle to get adequate protein that prevents loss of lean mass, people following this diet are typically not overweight. It's challenging to get a lot of energy from plant-based foods in their unrefined forms.

However, the problem with simply thinking in terms of plant-based vs animal-based foods is that most nutrient-poor, hyperpalatable foods found in the bottom-left corner of the satiety vs nutrient density chart also come from plants.

When we combine nutrient-poor refined fats, starches, and sugars, we get foods like doughnuts, croissants, cookies, and milk chocolate that use the hyperpalatable fat and carb combination to drive us into an uncontrollable feeding frenzy.

There is a practical limit to how many non-starchy veggies you can eat. You might feel like you're going to explode if you tried to get your daily energy requirements from watercress or spinach. So, once you've got your fill of greens, you need to wisely choose where to get your energy from by moving down the top right of the chart to more nutritious energy-dense foods. We tend to find that people with the best micronutrient profiles get their nutrients from a combination of plant-based foods, meat, and seafood.

The nutrient density vs satiety chart below shows the same data after removing vegetables, fruit, and spices. In the top right of this chart, we have seafood, dairy, and other animal-based foods. You can use these to simultaneously get adequate energy and nutrients.

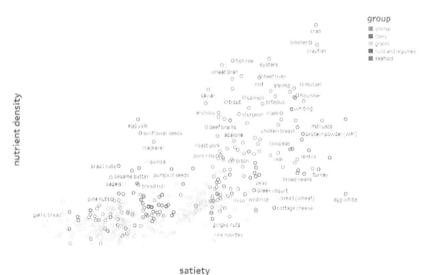

If you need more energy to support your activity and don't have weight to lose, you can include more energy-dense foods towards the bottom left corner. However, the sad reality is that most of us primarily eat low-satiety nutrient-poor foods found in the bottom left corner and would benefit from adding more foods located towards the top right.

The key thing to remember about Nutritional Optimisation is that it's a progressive process. Most people don't have lasting success when they change everything overnight.

In our Micros Masterclass, we initially guide people to review their current diet. Once they understand their baseline diet, they progressively add in more nutrient-dense foods and meals to plug their micronutrient gaps and drop the less optimal options that no longer fit.

Will Nutrient-Dense Foods Help Me Lose Weight?

Nutrient-dense foods and meals often provide greater satiety and allow us to consume less food without actively fighting our hunger.

The chart below shows our measure for diet quality, the Optimal Nutrient Intake Score (ONI), vs calorie intake that has been quantified from 125,761 days of macronutrient and micronutrient data from 34,519 people who have used Nutrient Optimiser to fine-tune their nutrition. As people level up their nutrient density, their cravings are satisfied, and they tend to eat less. So, once we dial in food quality, food quantity tends to look after itself!

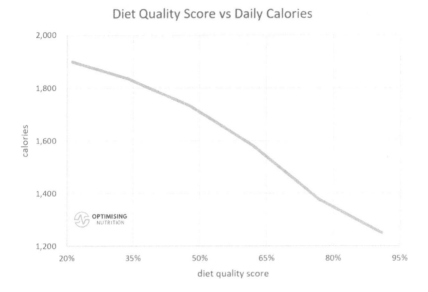

Diet Quality Score vs Daily Calories

The good news is that nutrient-dense foods and meals do not tend to contain refined carbs or seed oils. If you're focusing on maximising nutrient density, you won't be getting excessive amounts of refined carbohydrates or processed seed oils either. Once you learn to focus on nutrient density and satiety, balancing between carbs and fat becomes irrelevant.

Which Nutrients Do I Need More of to Help Me Eat Less?

Through our analysis of data from Optimisers, we have gained a fascinating insight into how different macronutrients and micronutrients influence our appetite and total caloric intake throughout the day.

In line with the Protein Leverage Hypothesis, our data shows that we eat less when a greater proportion of our diet comes from protein rather than fat and/or carbohydrates.

As shown in the chart below, people who consume a higher protein % tend to eat 55% fewer calories.

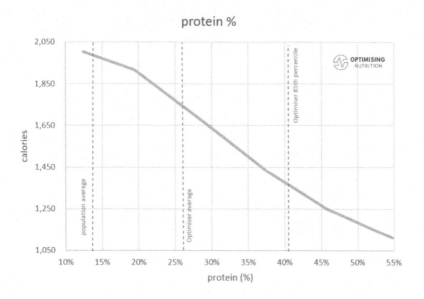

Conversely, the more energy we get from non-fibre carbohydrates and fat, the more we eat.

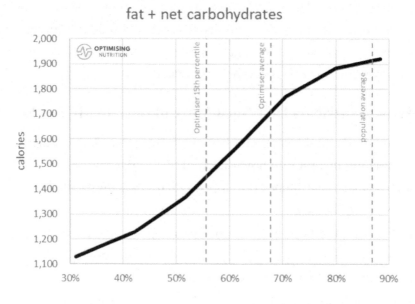

However, our data indicate that, rather than merely protein leverage, there is also a micronutrient leverage effect for each micronutrient. As a result, we tend to eat less when we consume foods that contain more of each micronutrient per calorie, as shown in the charts below.

After protein, potassium has the strongest satiety impact of all the micronutrients. People who consume foods with more potassium per calorie tend to eat 50% less!

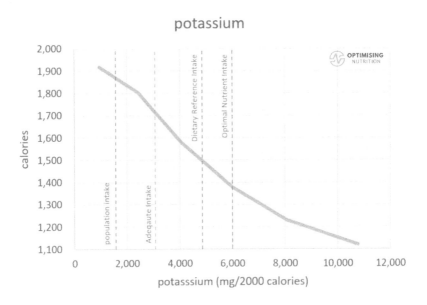

potassium

While some micronutrients continue to provide greater satiety with no upper limit in terms of nutrients per calorie, some nutrients like vitamins have a limited impact on satiety.

The data indicate that once we get enough of one particular nutrient, our appetite for these foods settles down, and we no longer crave foods that contain more of this nutrient. We then seek out foods rich in other nutrients.

You will see a 'stretch target', or the Optimal Nutrient Intake, on the charts. These are based on either:

- the amount of the nutrient where more doesn't provide further benefit.
- the amount that most people can obtain with food alone, or the 85th percentile intake based on Optimiser data.

The charts below show the satiety response curves with the
Optimal Nutrient Intake for each of the essential micronutrients.

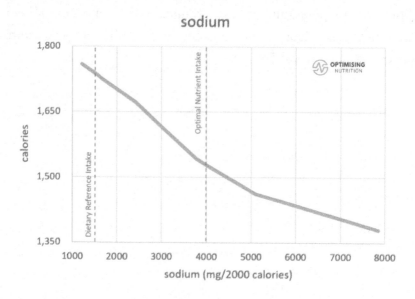

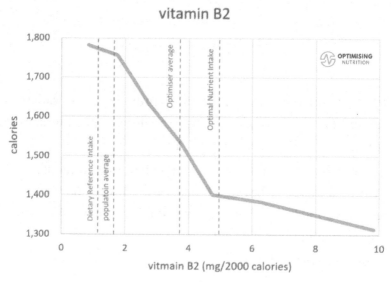

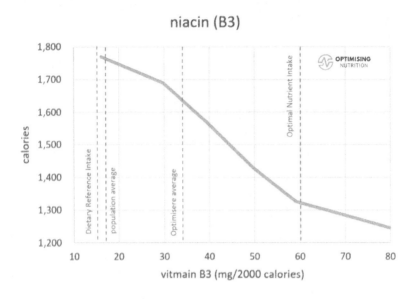

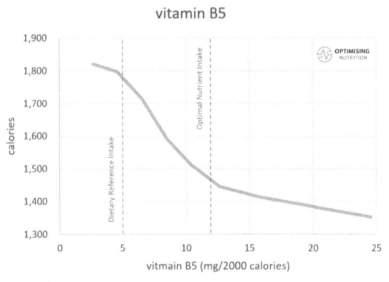

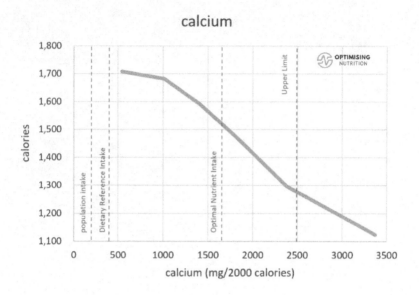

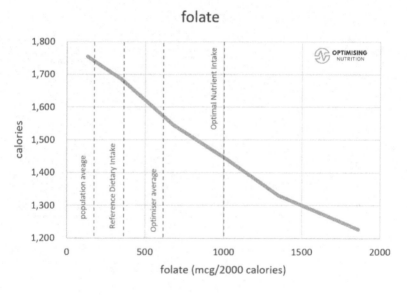

iron

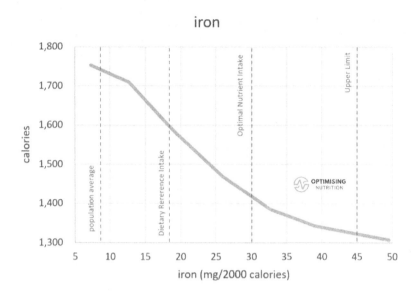

selenium

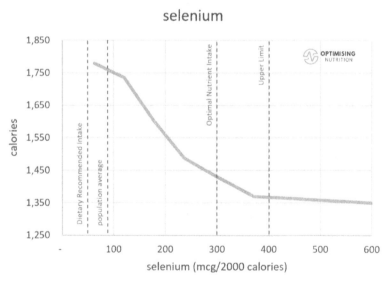

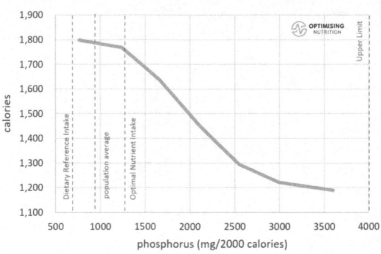

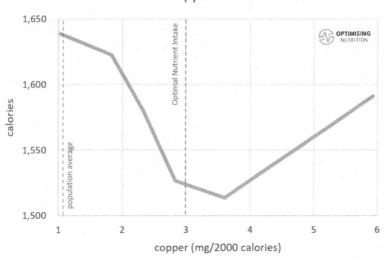

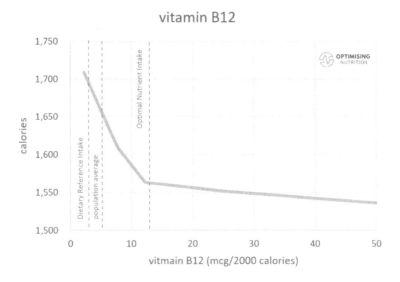

vitamin B12

What Does Each Nutrient Do for Us?

The functions and interactions of the micronutrients in our body
are complex, and we are only just coming to understand them.
A few highlights are noted below.

- **Vitamin C** is an antioxidant that protects the body from
  cardiovascular diseases, cancers, joint diseases, cataracts,
  and the common cold. It is necessary for collagen and
  elastin synthesis, which are necessary elements in the bone
  matrix, skin, tooth dentin, blood vessels, and tendons. It
  protects against oxygen-based damage to cells (free
  radicals or reactive oxygen species), is required for fat
  synthesis, and has antiviral and detoxifying properties.

- **Calcium** is needed for bone and tooth formation, muscle
  contraction, blood clotting, and nerve transmission. It also
  reduces the risk of colon cancer and prevents hypertension.

- **Chromium** assists with insulin function, helps lower
  elevated serum cholesterol and triglycerides and is required
  for carbohydrate and fat metabolism. It also increases
  fertility and is essential for fetal growth and development.

- **Copper** is necessary for bone formation, energy production, colouring of the hair and skin, and taste sensitivity. It is involved in collagen synthesis and the wound healing process. Copper also aids in iron transport and helps metabolise several fatty acids.
- **Magnesium** is involved in over 300 essential metabolic reactions. It is necessary for muscle activity and nerve impulses, regulating temperature and blood pressure, and it is essential for detoxification. Working with calcium, magnesium also helps to build strong bones and teeth.
- **Choline** is vital for lipid and cholesterol transport and metabolising of methyl groups. It also improves cognitive function and memory.
- **Potassium** is the major cation of intracellular fluid. It is an almost constant component of lean body tissues. The flux of potassium out of cells and sodium into cells changes the electrical potential during depolarisation and nerve and muscle cells' repolarisation. This process is helpful for nerve signalling and ATP production.
- **Selenium** is an antioxidant and is essential in redox reactions. It also is an important nutrient for the immune system and thyroid metabolism.
- **Phosphorus** is the second most abundant inorganic element in the body. Phosphorus as phosphate works as a significant buffer and helps to protect and balance blood pH. Phosphorus is critical to energy transfer in your body, including the generation of adenosine triphosphate (ATP).
- **Vitamin B12** is required to synthesise fatty acids in myelin and works in conjunction with folate to synthesise DNA and neurotransmitters. Adequate vitamin B12 intake is essential for healthy blood cells and neurological function. B12 is one of the main nutrients that drive the process

known as methylation.

- **Sodium** is the primary cation in human extracellular fluid. It is essential for maintaining critical physiological activities like extracellular fluid volume and cellular membrane potential.

For more details, check out our detailed articles on each of the micronutrients:

- Calcium
- Iron
- Magnesium
- Phosphorus
- Potassium
- Sodium
- Zinc
- Selenium
- Copper
- Manganese
- Vitamin A
- Vitamin E
- Thiamine (B1)
- Riboflavin (B2)
- Niacin (B3)
- Pantothenic acid (B5)
- Vitamin B6
- Folate (B9)
- Vitamin B12
- Vitamin C
- Vitamin D
- Choline
- Vitamin K1
- Omega 3

Can I Just Take a Pill?

People buy expensive supplements and pills in hopes of an easy fix for their otherwise nutrient-poor diet.

There is not a lot of money in nutrient-dense whole foods, so there isn't much advertising budget behind the #foodfirst message.

But if you stop and think for a second, when was the last time you saw someone get healthy by taking a 'magic pill' without changing their diet or activity?

While there may be some benefits from vitamin pills and food fortification, supplements are often not in the form the body needs, nor are they found in the synergistic ratios found in whole foods.

It's also likely you're not just missing one nutrient but rather a suite of beneficial compounds working in tandem that come from eating whole foods. In all honesty, we don't fully understand many of these nutrients quite yet.

Most studies have shown limited value in supplementing synthetic nutrient isolates unless there is a clear-cut clinical deficiency. However, countless studies have shown the innumerable benefits that come from eating nutrient-dense whole foods.

While supplements seem like an attractive option, they often don't provide the same benefit when separated from whole foods. Because nutrients work alongside one another, they can also drive nutrient imbalances.

The Optimal Nutrient Intakes

Current Recommendations

You may have heard of the Dietary Reference Intakes (DRI), which are set to prevent diseases of deficiency, or the Adequate Intakes (AI), which are calculated from typical population intakes when not enough studies are available to demonstrate a minimum level.

The Upper Limits (UL) are found based on the quantities of nutrients in their refined supplemental forms that are known to produce adverse symptoms in some people. Excess or overdose of nutrients is rarely a concern from whole foods.

But similar to protein targets, these recommended intake levels should be seen as a *minimum* as they are designed to avoid deficiency and not to ensure an *optimal* outcome. They are set in the context of the current food system, which has been optimised to feed a growing population in a cost-effective manner that focuses on food products that are produced most easily and not most healthily.

Your Nutritional Factor of Safety

In engineering, we work to find the balance between safety and cost by applying a factor of safety.

You probably wouldn't feel safe driving a truck across a bridge if you knew it had been designed for the absolute minimum cost. Even though engineers have undertaken many tests and have been using materials like steel and concrete for a long time, there are still many unknowns.

In geotechnical design, things are hard to test because they are under the ground and hard to see and clearly understand. Thus, we must apply a higher and more conservative factor of safety.

Designing a road or bridge slightly stronger than the absolute minimum ensures that it is resilient and won't be destroyed by extraordinary events and collapse catastrophically (e.g., an overloaded truck, an earthquake or a significant flood).

In a similar way, we can apply a larger factor of safety to our nutrient intake targets as we have for our Optimal Nutrient Intakes (ONIs). There are still many unknowns and things we don't understand when it comes to how your body uses the various nutrients in different circumstances.

We increase our nutritional safety factor by ensuring we are getting more than the absolute minimum nutrient intake. Rather than the bare minimum to prevent disease and death, we provide our body with higher quality building blocks that increase its resiliency and ability to cope with more stress and unforeseen extreme events.

We designed our Optimal Nutrient Intakes (ONIs) stretch targets based on the intakes that provide the greatest satiety. Aiming for the ONIs will help you reverse (or avoid) energy toxicity while still getting plenty of the essential nutrients you need to optimise mitochondrial function and metabolic health.

These are definitely stretch targets that are a challenge to achieve for most! However, we have seen numerous participants in our Micros Masterclass achieve *all* of them *at once* and reach an ONI score of 100% using Nutrient Optimiser, which guides people to obtain more of the nutrients their current diet lacks.

To get a taste for what nutrient density looks like in practice, see *What Do Top Optimisers Eat Across the Globe?*

Macronutrients

The chart below compares the satiety impact of each macronutrient based on our data analysis.

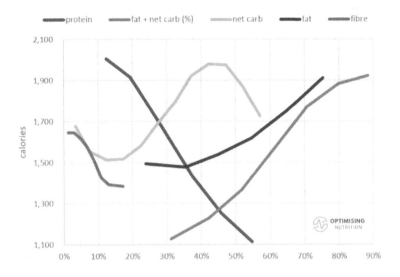

While fibre has a positive effect on satiety, most people don't consume enough of it to see a significant effect. Protein has the largest positive impact on satiety, while carbs and fat negatively impact satiety.

The table below shows macronutrient ranges that align with greater satiety and nutrient density. Notice how there is plenty of room for movement within these ranges to find the macro split that suits your goals and preferences.

Macronutrient	Range
Protein	< 50%
Net carbs	10 – 45%
Fat	> 30%

We don't recommend immediately jumping straight to these stretch targets. In our Macros Masterclass, we guide people to assess their current typical macronutrient profile and make progressive tweaks to move towards their goals in a sustainable manner.

Minerals

Adequate mineral intake is critical! But in comparison to vitamins, minerals are bulky. Thus, they are rarely provided in adequate quantities through supplements or food fortification. Instead, you *must* get your minerals from nutrient-dense food!

The comparison chart below shows that all minerals positively impact satiety. However, calcium, phosphorus, magnesium, potassium, sodium, and zinc have the most significant impacts (i.e., the longer the line, the greater the impact).

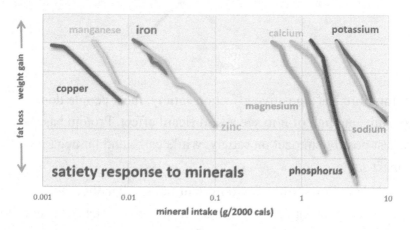

Vitamins

Foods that contain more vitamins tend to be more satiating, but only up to a point. There appears to be a level beyond what nutrient-dense whole foods can provide for most vitamins where there is no additional benefit, at least in terms of satiety.

Big Fat Keto Lies

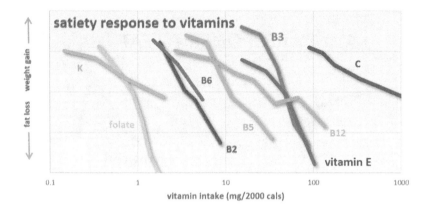

While the ONIs for vitamins are typically around six times the minimum Recommended Dietary Allowances, higher levels only achievable through supplementation don't provide additional benefits.

Unless you have a measured clinical deficiency of a particular nutrient, adding more vitamins into your system above the ONIs likely just creates expensive, brightly coloured pee!

Fatty Acids

Fat is a controversial macronutrient. Generally, higher intakes of fat do not tend to be satiating. However, our analysis also identified that:

- your ratio of Omega-6 to Omega-3 fatty acids is important, and most people should increase their intake of seafood and avoid foods that contain refined seed oils.
- if you want to lose weight, focusing on reducing your monounsaturated fat intake from added oils or as processed food ingredients will give you the biggest bang for your buck; and
- you needn't worry about nutritious foods that naturally contain cholesterol, saturated fat, or even trans fats.

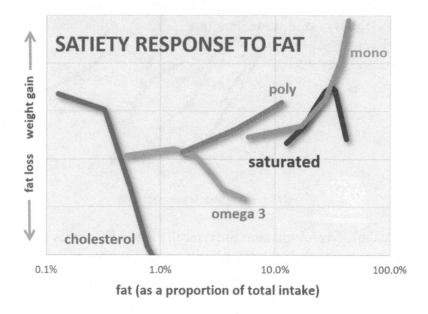

Amino Acids

Each amino acid has a unique biological function. Different protein sources like fish, eggs, meat, offal, beans, and legumes each have their own unique amino acid profiles.

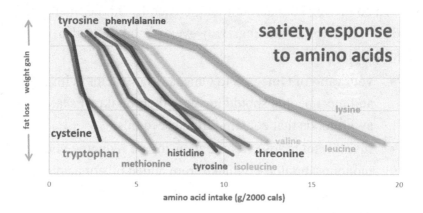

While you'll probably hit your protein and amino acid targets with whole protein sources, the table below shows recommended stretch targets for each amino acid.

What Are the Optimal Nutrient Intakes?

The <u>Optimal Nutrient Intakes (ONIs)</u>, shown in the table below, are the quantities of each nutrient our data has shown to align with consistently greater satiety and optimised health.

nutrient	ONI	DRI or AI	units
calcium	1650	1000	mg
iron	30	18	mg
magnesium	825	320	mg
phosphorus	1250	700	mg
potassium	6000	2600	mg
sodium	4000	1500	mg
zinc	25	8.0	mg
copper	3	0.9	mg
manganese	5.5	1.8	mg
selenium	300	55	mcg
vitamin A	10000	2333	IU
vitamin E	25	15	mg
vitamin D	1200	600	IU
vitamin C	350	75	mg
thiamine (B1)	3	1.1	mg
riboflavin (B2)	6	1.1	mg
niacin (B3)	60	14	mg
pantothenic acid (B5)	12	5	mg
vitamin B6	5	1.3	mg
vitamin B12	12	2.4	mcg
vitamin K1	1100	90	mcg
folate	1000	400	mcg
tryptophan	2.2	-	g
threonine	8.1	-	g

nutrient	ONI	DRI or AI	units
isoleucine	8.8	-	g
leucine	15.2	-	g
lysine	15.2	-	g
methionine	4.8	-	g
cysteine	2.4	0.9	g
phenylalanine	7.9	1.6	g
tyrosine	6.6	1.6	g
valine	9.8	2.3	g
histidine	5.4	1.4	g
omega 3	6	1.1	g

Also shown for comparison are the DRIs and Ais, which are calculated based on the average intake of a 70 kg man who theoretically consumes 2000 calories per day. The ONIs shown in this table are based on 2000 calories per day for ease of comparison.

On average, the ONIs are around *four times* the DRI, or AI required to prevent diseases of deficiency. If you're aiming for the ONI targets and are eating in a calorie deficit to lose weight, you will still be getting plenty of these nutrients.

How Can I Level Up from the DRIs to ONIs?

Because the minimum nutrient intakes are low, many people find it reasonably easy to reach them in Cronometer and see lots of green straight away. However, they get discouraged when they start by putting the ONI stretch targets shown in the table above into Cronometer, and all their pretty green bars turn yellow and shrink.

Nutrient Targets

General				Vitamins			
Energy	1913.4	kcal	98%	B1 (Thiamine)	1.1	mg	
				B2 (Riboflavin)	4.2	mg	323%
Carbohydrates				B3 (Niacin)	51.1	mg	319%
Fiber	20.7	g	54%	B5 (Pantothenic Acid)	28.9	mg	579%
Net Carbs	69.6	g	73%	B6 (Pyridoxine)	5.6	mg	428%
				B12 (Cobalamin)	39.4	µg	1641%
Lipids				Folate	405.1	µg	101%
Fat	85.4	g	90%	Vitamin A	15367.2	IU	512%
				Vitamin C	78.0	mg	87%
Protein				Vitamin D	550.3	IU	92%
Protein	193.7	g	105%	Vitamin E	9.3	mg	62%
Cystine	2.5	g	282%	Vitamin K	325.0	µg	271%
Glycine	6.9	g	174%				
Histidine	4.5	g	320%	Minerals			
Isoleucine	8.5	g	440%	Calcium	1122.1	mg	112%
Leucine	14.5	g	341%	Copper	2.3	mg	255%
Lysine	13.8	g	358%	Iron	22.3	mg	278%
Methionine	4.2	g	441%	Magnesium	453.4	mg	108%
Phenylalanine	7.5	g	451%	Manganese	2.9	mg	125%
Threonine	8.0	g	395%	Phosphorus	2041.8	mg	292%
Tryptophan	2.2	g	432%	Potassium	4381.3	mg	123%
Tyrosine	6.1	g	368%	Selenium	221.4	µg	403%
Valine	9.5	g	392%	Sodium	3352.0	mg	223%
				Zinc	19.6	mg	179%

The "beginner" column in the table below shows the DRI/AIs that you will see in <u>Cronometer</u> by default. In addition, we have the ONI targets per 2000 calories (i.e., Level 3).

If you want to work your way up to the ONI targets in 'digestible' phases, you can start by changing your settings in <u>Cronometer</u> to the ONIs per 1000 calories (i.e. Level 1). This will highlight the nutrients you need to focus on more effectively.

Meanwhile, anything that is still green and full in Cronometer is good to go – you are already getting plenty of these nutrients. These Level 1 targets are handy for people consuming fewer calories in a weight loss phase or older females who require fewer calories than active young men.

nutrient	Beginner DRI/AI	Level 1 ONI (1000 cals)	Level 2 ONI (1500 cals)	Level 3 ONI (2000 cals)
calcium	1000	825	1,238	1650
iron	18	15	23	30
magnesium	320	412.5	619	825
phosphorus	700	625	938	1250
potassium	2600	3000	4,500	6000
sodium	1500	2000	3,000	4000
zinc	8	12.5	19	25
copper	0.9	1.5	2.3	3
manganese	1.8	2.75	4.1	5.5
selenium	55	150	225	300
vitamin A	2333	5000	7,500	10000
vitamin E	15	12.5	19	25
vitamin D	600	600	900	1200
vitamin C	75	175	263	350
thiamine (B1)	1.1	1.5	2.3	3
riboflavin (B2)	1.1	3	4.5	6
niacin (B3)	14	30	45	60
vitamin B5	5	6	9	12
vitamin B6	1.3	2.5	3.8	5
vitamin (B12)	2.4	6	9	12
vitamin K1	90	550	825	1100
folate	400	500	750	1000
tryptophan	0	1.1	1.7	2.2
threonine	0	4.1	6.1	8.1
isoleucine	0	4.4	6.6	8.8
leucine	0	7.6	11.4	15.2
lysine	0	7.6	11.4	15.2
methionine	0	2.4	3.6	4.8
cysteine	0.9	1.2	1.8	2.4
phenylalanine	1.6	4.0	5.9	7.9
tyrosine	1.6	3.3	5.0	6.6
valine	2.3	4.9	7.4	9.8

nutrient	Beginner DRI/AI	Level 1 ONI (1000 cals)	Level 2 ONI (1500 cals)	Level 3 ONI (2000 cals)
histidine	1.4	2.7	4.1	5.4
omega 3	1.1	3.0	4.5	6.0

Then, once you are getting full green bars for most of the nutrients with the Level 1 targets, you can enter the ONIs per 1500 calories (Level 2) and continue focusing on nutrients that are harder to find. Finally, if you eat around 2000 calories and mainly see green bars, you can level up to the ONI per 2000 calorie targets.

Updating your nutrient targets in Cronometer won't change anything in Nutrient Optimiser. It simply makes the display in Cronometer a little more helpful and motivational as you continue on your quest toward Nutritional Optimisation.

For more details on this process, see The Nutrient Bucket-Filling Game.

Which Nutrients Do YOU Need More of?

People often ask what the most nutrient-dense diet, meals, and foods are. Unfortunately, the answer depends on *your* goals and *your* current diet. While we have created nutrient-dense foods and recipes to contain more of the nutrients that most people struggle to get enough of, nutrient density should ideally be tailored to an individual's diet and goals.

To demonstrate, the following sections look at the nutrient profiles of several different dietary approaches.

The Hardest Nutrients to Find in our Food System

The nutrient fingerprint chart below shows the nutrient profiles for over 9,000 commonly available foods that are listed on the USDA Food Composition Database.

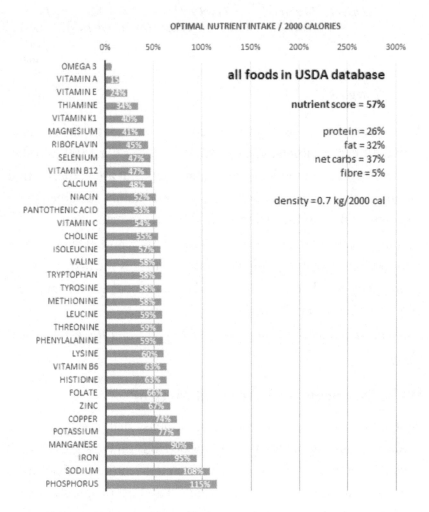

OPTIMAL NUTRIENT INTAKE / 2000 CALORIES

all foods in USDA database

nutrient score = 57%

protein = 26%
fat = 32%
net carbs = 37%
fibre = 5%

density = 0.7 kg/2000 cal

As a general rule, we will struggle to get enough omega-3 fatty acids, vitamin A, vitamin E, thiamine (B1), and other nutrients listed towards the top of this chart.

Plant-Based Foods

The micronutrient fingerprint chart below shows the nutrient profile if we just went 'plant-based' without considering nutrient density.

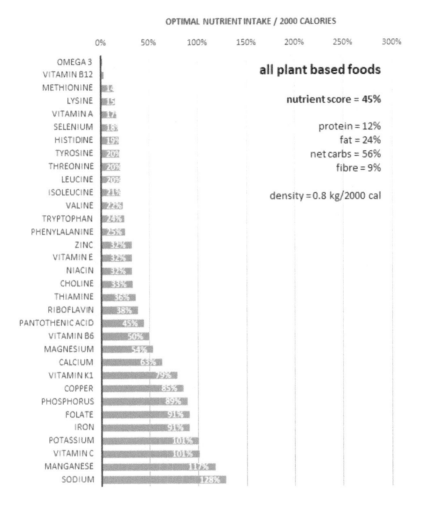

OPTIMAL NUTRIENT INTAKE / 2000 CALORIES

all plant based foods

nutrient score = 45%

protein = 12%
fat = 24%
net carbs = 56%
fibre = 9%

density = 0.8 kg/2000 cal

The good news is we can boost the nutrients in a purely plant-based diet by focusing on foods containing more of the harder-to-find nutrients towards the top of the nutrient fingerprint chart.

The micronutrient fingerprint chart below shows the nutrient profile of the most nutrient-dense plant-based foods. As you can see, someone strictly following a plant-based diet may still struggle to get enough vitamin B12, omega-3, selenium, vitamin A, and certain amino acids.

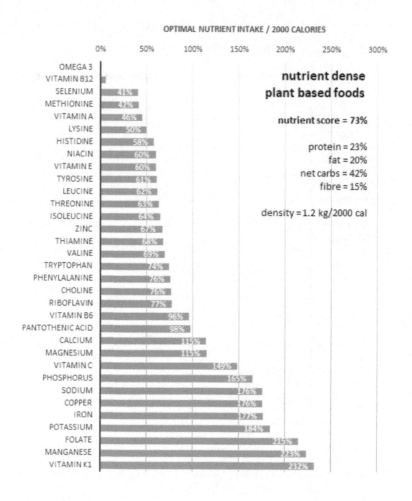

OPTIMAL NUTRIENT INTAKE / 2000 CALORIES

**nutrient dense
plant based foods**

nutrient score = 73%

protein = 23%
fat = 20%
net carbs = 42%
fibre = 15%

density = 1.2 kg/2000 cal

But as the chart shows below, the nutrient profile could sadly be much worse if a 'plant-based diet' merely means eliminating animal products without prioritising the required nutrients through vegetables, nuts, and seeds. There is plenty of 'plant-based' vegan junk food that mostly combines low-satiety, nutrient-poor processed oils, sugar, and refined grains.

So, if you choose to follow a plant-based diet, you should make a special effort to prioritise minimally processed foods like vegetables and seeds while minimising refined oils and processed grains.

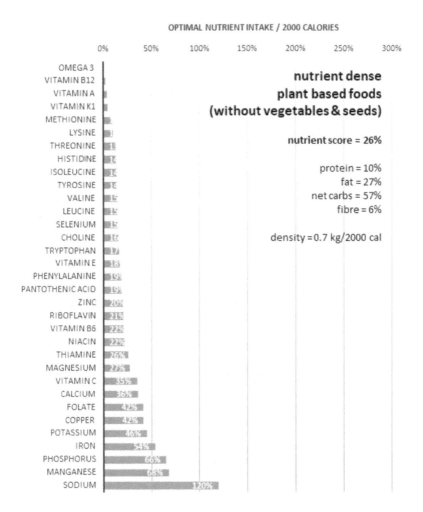

OPTIMAL NUTRIENT INTAKE / 2000 CALORIES

nutrient dense
plant based foods
(without vegetables & seeds)

nutrient score = 26%

protein = 10%
fat = 27%
net carbs = 57%
fibre = 6%

density = 0.7 kg/2000 cal

Animal-Based Foods

Meanwhile, someone on a carnivore diet at the other end of the dietary spectrum may struggle to get enough vitamin K1, vitamin C, folate, or other nutrients found towards the top of this chart.

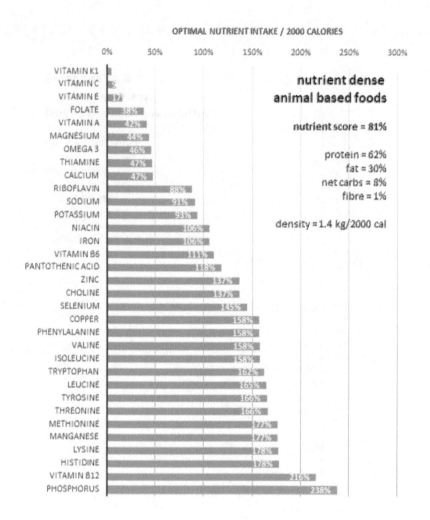

OPTIMAL NUTRIENT INTAKE / 2000 CALORIES

nutrient dense
animal based foods

nutrient score = 81%

protein = 62%
fat = 30%
net carbs = 8%
fibre = 1%

density = 1.4 kg/2000 cal

Can I Get Too Much of a Good Thing?

It's difficult to get too much of any of the micronutrients from whole foods alone. Your kidneys do an excellent job of filtering out excess nutrients that you don't require.

As you can see from the satiety response curves above, we benefit from consuming nutrients well above the recommended minimum intake levels *when they come from whole foods*.

There are some anecdotal cases of Arctic explorers consuming too much polar bear liver and feeling ill from hypervitaminosis A. But in practice, most people don't eat excessive amounts of liver, let alone from polar bears when they are dehydrated.

It is possible, however, to overdo your supplements. In the first instance, excessive supplementation can give you diarrhea as your body sheds them from your system. There are also many instances where excessive levels of one nutrient can affect the absorption of other nutrients because of the synergistic and antagonistic relationships to one another, which can create severe issues.

While a multivitamin probably won't hurt you, you should ideally understand why you are taking it and use it as a supplement to make up for the nutrients you know you're not getting from whole food because you're tracking your diet.

You should also be aware that nutrients in whole foods come in the forms and ratios that your body needs and recognises. Nutrients don't act alone, and each nutrient works synergistically with other nutrients.

The good news is that, as you start to dial in your nutrient density in the food you eat, you will quickly find that you no longer need to rely on supplements, and you can save your money to invest in quality food.

For more details, see Micronutrient Balance Ratios: Do They Matter and How Can I Manage Them?

Bioavailability

Plant-based foods often contain more concentrated quantities of certain nutrients per calorie. However, the nutrients in animal foods tend to be more 'bioavailable', meaning they're in forms that are easily used in the body.

For example, the forms of vitamin A, iron, and omega-3 fatty acids found in animal foods are already in the most active forms for the body and do not require any conversion. In contrast, plant-based foods contain nutrient *precursors*, meaning the nutrients need to be converted before the body can use them.

There are some losses in the conversion of nutrients, and some people are better than others at converting for various reasons like stress and genetics. As a result, the number of nutrients in plant-based foods doesn't equate to nutrients in the body.

Unfortunately, there is not a lot of reliable data to quantify how much of the nutrients are converted. At the same time, less bioavailable nutrients like beta carotene, the precursor to vitamin A found in fruits and vegetables, are generally relatively easy to get in adequate quantities. Although there is uncertainty around bioavailability, it doesn't stop us from using the data we do have to optimise your diet!

While it would be great to have accurate data to quantify the losses that occur during the conversion of precursors from plant-based foods vs the bioavailable nutrients found in animal-based foods, it doesn't have a significant consequence if you are focusing on a range of nutrient-dense foods.

Your metabolism is highly complex, and there is a LOT we still don't understand about how it works. But, if you give your body all the nutrients it needs in the forms it recognises, there is a pretty good chance it will know what to do with them.

We recommend you prioritise foods that contain more nutrients that align with your goals. Whether you eat more non-starchy vegetables, more organ meats, more seafood, or more meat, it doesn't matter because you will be making significant improvements compared to a diet of refined grains and oils.

If you are still concerned about bioavailability down the track, you can look at the micronutrient fingerprint of the foods you eat most often. If there are nutrients you find harder to get enough of at the top of your micronutrient fingerprint that are not bioavailable from the foods you're eating, you can prioritise more bioavailable sources of those nutrients. But this is getting into the weeds, and most people don't need to be concerned about this level of minutiae.

To identify your priority micronutrients and which foods and meals will fill the gaps, you can use our 7-day Nutrient Clarity Challenge.

What About Anti-Nutrients?

Plant-based foods like grains and legumes contain 'anti-nutrients' like lectins, phytic acid, goitrogens, oxalates, and tannins that can hinder the absorption of nutrients such as calcium, zinc, iron, magnesium, and potassium.

For people who have a history of digestive problems, lectins are often an issue. These compounds are found readily in vegetables, beans, legumes, and grains and can activate the immune system and contribute to intestinal permeability ('leaky gut').

Grain-based foods are not only relatively nutrient-poor, but they also contain some of the most concentrated amounts of antinutrients like phytic acid, lectins, and oxalate. All of these compounds inhibit the absorption of other essential nutrients.

There are some substances in vegetables like sulforaphane that are considered to be antinutrients. However, some people see these as positive because they provide beneficial hormetic stress that strengthens your system, similar to the way resistance training builds strength.

If your digestion isn't great, you may benefit from an autoimmune elimination diet (AIP) or even a carnivorous diet for a time to see your symptoms improve. When you are symptom free, you can progressively reintroduce the most nutrient-dense foods and see how your body responds.

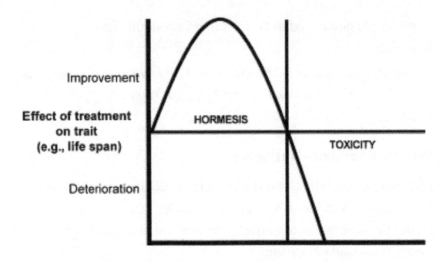

Focusing on nutrient-dense foods and meals means you automatically minimise anti-nutrients because they are free from refined grains that contain most of the antinutrients in our food system.

The remaining ones in vegetables don't appear to be significant issue for most people without pre-existing conditions. If you have specific symptoms or digestive problems when you eat certain foods, it may pay to listen to your body and reduce them.

There's no point in eating foods that give you digestive upset. But eliminating all plant foods because they are 'out to get you' may leave you with a super fragile digestive system. Over time, you want to build resilience in *all* areas of your body.

Nutrients in Low-Carb Foods vs High-Fat Foods

Many people following a ketogenic or low-carb diet think in terms of their food as either 'low-carb' or 'high-fat'. Let's look at the nutritional implications of thinking in terms of these extremes.

Nutrients in Low-Carb Foods

The nutrient fingerprint chart below shows the nutrient content of the lowest carb foods in the USDA database.

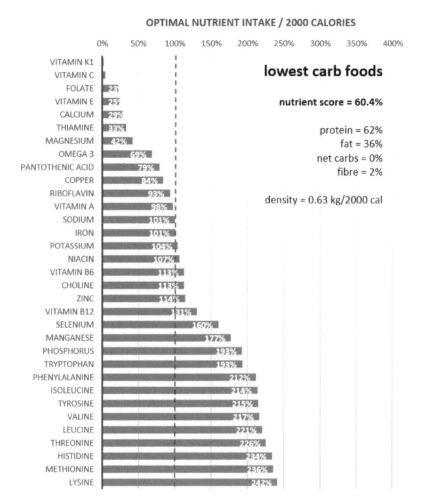

OPTIMAL NUTRIENT INTAKE / 2000 CALORIES

lowest carb foods

nutrient score = 60.4%

protein = 62%
fat = 36%
net carbs = 0%
fibre = 2%

density = 0.63 kg/2000 cal

Nutrient	%
VITAMIN K1	
VITAMIN C	
FOLATE	23%
VITAMIN E	25%
CALCIUM	29%
THIAMINE	33%
MAGNESIUM	42%
OMEGA 3	69%
PANTOTHENIC ACID	79%
COPPER	84%
RIBOFLAVIN	93%
VITAMIN A	98%
SODIUM	101%
IRON	101%
POTASSIUM	104%
NIACIN	107%
VITAMIN B6	113%
CHOLINE	113%
ZINC	114%
VITAMIN B12	131%
SELENIUM	160%
MANGANESE	177%
PHOSPHORUS	193%
TRYPTOPHAN	193%
PHENYLALANINE	212%
ISOLEUCINE	214%
TYROSINE	215%
VALINE	217%
LEUCINE	221%
THREONINE	226%
HISTIDINE	234%
METHIONINE	236%
LYSINE	242%

The horizontal axis represents the percentage of the Optimal Nutrient Intake per 2000 calories. The nutrient score is based on the area to the left of the 100% Optimal Nutrient Intake (ONI) and is represented as the red dotted line.

On the upside, these very low-carb foods contain heaps of bioavailable protein, which is likely a big reason why many people do so well when starting a low-carb diet. However, the downside is that these foods lack essential nutrients shown at the top like vitamin K1, vitamin C, folate, calcium, magnesium, and omega-3 fatty acids.

In comparison, the micronutrient fingerprint shown below represents the highest fat foods.

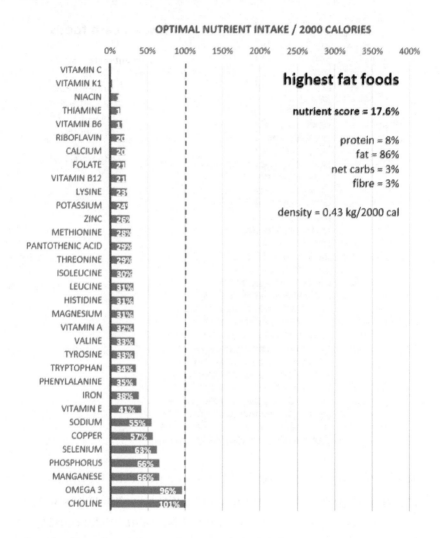

OPTIMAL NUTRIENT INTAKE / 2000 CALORIES

highest fat foods

nutrient score = 17.6%

protein = 8%
fat = 86%
net carbs = 3%
fibre = 3%

density = 0.43 kg/2000 cal

When both carbs and protein are minimised, we get a poor overall nutrient profile that is much worse than the lowest carbohydrate foods. So, when it comes to getting enough nutrients from the food you eat, it seems low-carb prevails over high fat.

Finally, we have the nutrient fingerprint of the foods with the highest nutrient density. If you only ate these foods, you would get all the nutrients you need quickly. They are also extraordinarily satiating and hard to overeat, meaning your body would likely produce endogenous ketones from your stored fat if you stayed below your calorie parameter.

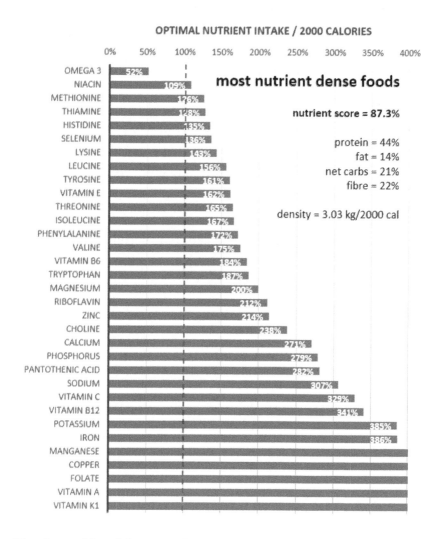

The downside of these foods is that they are hard to get enough energy from. Thus, it can be wise to progressively 'level up' your diet based on your current situation and goals. For weight loss, you can progressively add in some more nutrient-dense foods and meals while dropping less optimal options. Conversely, to gain weight, while you should still prioritise nutrient density, you will also need some less nutrient-dense foods that contain energy from fat and/or carbs.

Our Nutrient-Dense Recipe Books

After trying to promote the benefits of focusing on <u>nutrient density</u> for years, we realised that we had to create some easy-to-make recipes that would enable people to bring the theory to life in their own kitchens.

Allow me to give you a tour through the nutrient profile of a few of our recipe books to show you what this looks like in practice as we apply nutritional optimisation for different contexts and goals.

Therapeutic keto

Our book of <u>recipes for therapeutic ketosis</u> is designed to help people achieve therapeutic ketone levels to manage epilepsy, dementia, or Parkinson's.

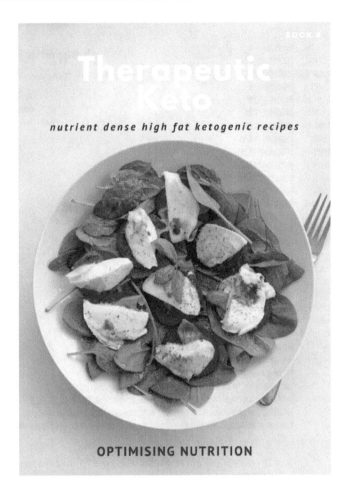

nutrient dense high fat ketogenic recipes

OPTIMISING NUTRITION

As you can see from the nutrient profile shown below, these recipes have plenty of fat and lower protein and a nutrient score of 48%. These charts for the recipe books are shown in terms of the Dietary Reference Intake per 2000 calories. With a high-fat therapeutic ketogenic diet, we can meet the minimum nutrient intake to prevent diseases of deficiency, although calcium and niacin (shown towards the top of the nutrient fingerprint chart) are still a challenge.

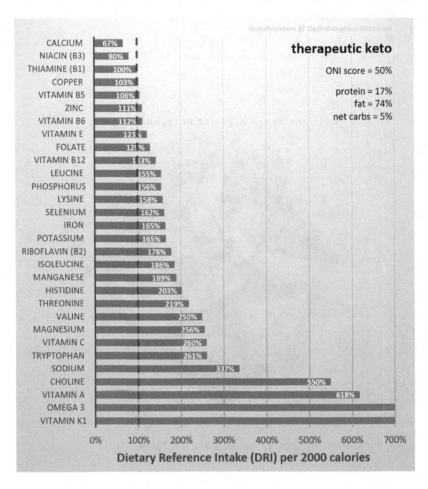

Let's use a hypothetical example of someone who weighs 70 kg with 20% body fat (i.e., lean body mass = 56 kg) who has a maintenance calorie intake of 2000 calories per day, who needs to gain weight (e.g., someone who needs to gain weight after cancer treatment or a child who has epilepsy who needed to grow).

The table below shows their intake in terms of calories, protein and net carbs if they ate these meals to different degrees of energy surplus.

surplus	diet (cals)	protein (g)	net carb (g)	protein (g/kg LBM)
0%	2000	65	25	1.2
10%	2200	72	28	1.3
20%	2400	78	30	1.4
30%	2600	85	33	1.5

They would be getting a moderate amount of protein without excess carbs, which would allow endogenous ketosis. The fact these foods are not exceptionally nutrient-dense wouldn't be a significant concern because they are eating a lot more calories and hence getting a reasonable amount of nutrients.

While the nutrient content is not optimal, this is not as big of a concern because exogenous ketosis is the highest priority. When eating these foods in a surplus, they would be getting adequate amounts of protein to support lean muscle mass while still allowing ketosis.

Nutritional Keto

The book is designed for someone who enjoys a ketogenic way of eating (without therapeutic ketone levels) and who doesn't necessarily have fat-loss goals.

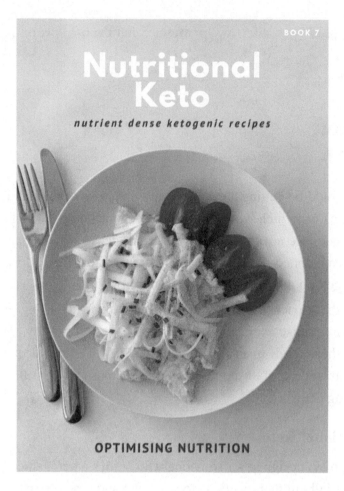

These recipes would be ideal for someone who is active and needs some extra energy to prevent weight loss.

These nutritional keto recipes have a higher nutrient density than the therapeutic keto approach, with more protein and less fat (although we still struggle to get the minimum intake of calcium and vitamin B1).

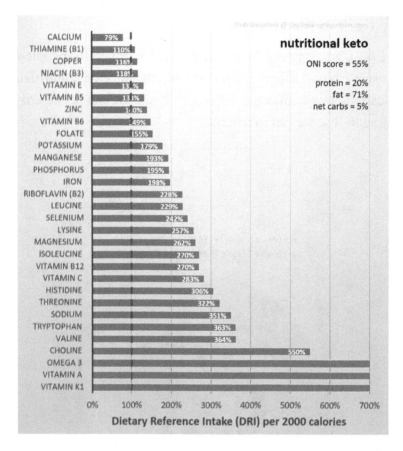

Let's say the person eating these meals is lean and already active and needs to eat in an energy surplus to support their activity. They would be getting adequate protein without excessive levels of carbohydrates. These meals also have a lower satiety value which would allow them to consume more energy to support their activity.

surplus	diet (cals)	net carb (g)	protein (g/kg LBM)
0%	2000	35	1.8
10%	2200	39	2.0
20%	2400	42	2.1
30%	2600	46	2.3

Low-Carb & Blood Sugar

Our Low Carb & Blood Sugar recipes are designed for people who want stable blood sugars and weight maintenance on a nutritious low-carb diet, who may not be as active, and are not necessarily wanting to lose weight in a hurry.

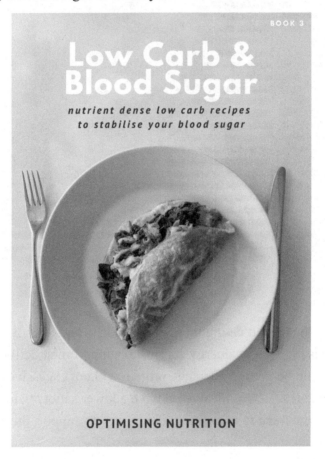

The recipes contain a substantial amount of protein and have a higher nutrient density score while still low in carbohydrates. We can meet the minimum nutrient intake with a low-carbohydrate diet optimised for healthy blood sugar levels.

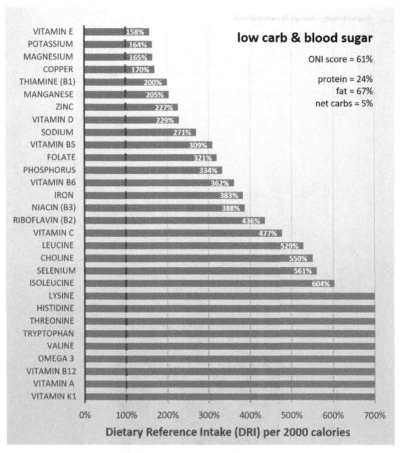

low carb & blood sugar

ONI score = 61%

protein = 24%
fat = 67%
net carbs = 5%

Dietary Reference Intake (DRI) per 2000 calories

If they ate these recipes for most of their meals and added some higher fat snacks, they would still be getting plenty of protein while keeping daily carbohydrate intake low to maintain stable blood sugar while also getting plenty of nutrients.

deficit	diet (cals)	body fat (cals)	net carb (g)	protein (g/kg LBM)
-10%	2200	-200	44	3.0
0%	2000	0	40	2.8
10%	1800	200	36	2.5
20%	1600	400	32	2.2
30%	1400	600	28	1.9

Blood sugar & fat loss

The <u>blood sugar and fat loss recipes</u> are ideal for anyone with elevated blood sugars and body fat to lose, as many people who find themselves diagnosed with Type 2 Diabetes tend to be.

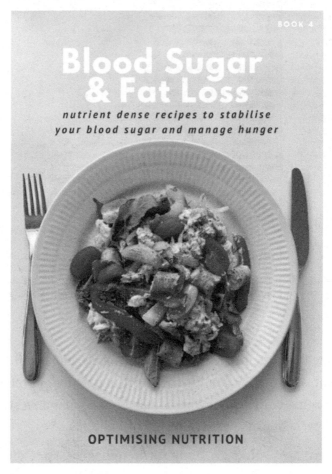

These recipes have a higher protein percentage for satiety and a greater <u>nutrient density</u> while still being lower in carbohydrates. They contain a moderate amount of fat, but if you are losing fat from your body, you will likely still be in (endogenous) ketosis, with some of the ketones coming from your body (rather than your diet).

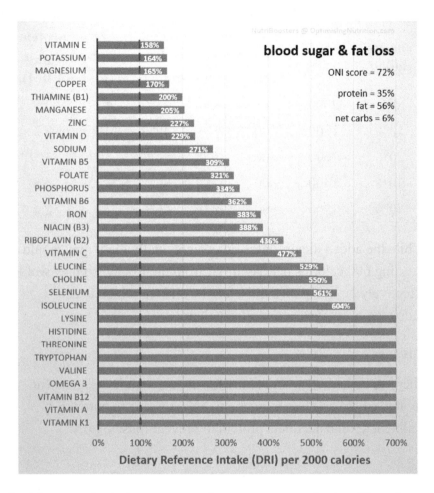

In this scenario, let's assume we have someone who has Type 2 Diabetes. They have started their low-carb or keto journey to stabilise their blood sugars, but they still have a lot of body fat to lose.

As we can see in the table below, it would be quite hard to eat enough of these meals due to the high-satiety effect of protein. Most people struggle to consume more than around 2.8 g/kg LBM of protein, so they would likely end up in a 30% energy deficit without having to watch their calories.

energy deficit	diet (cals)	body fat (cals)	total fat (cals)	total fat (%)	net carb (g)	protein (g/kg LBM)
0%	2000	0	860	43%	45	3.9
10%	1800	200	974	49%	41	3.5
20%	1600	400	1088	54%	36	3.1
30%	1400	600	1202	60%	32	2.8
40%	1200	800	1316	66%	27	2.4

While the added dietary fat is not exceptionally high, they would be using 600 calories per day of fat from their body, so they would effectively be living on a 60% fat diet and would likely see endogenous ketones coming from their body.

Fat loss

Then we have the Fat loss NutriBoosters, which is designed for greater satiety and less hunger and cravings due to nutrient deficiencies and adequate protein to prevent muscle loss.

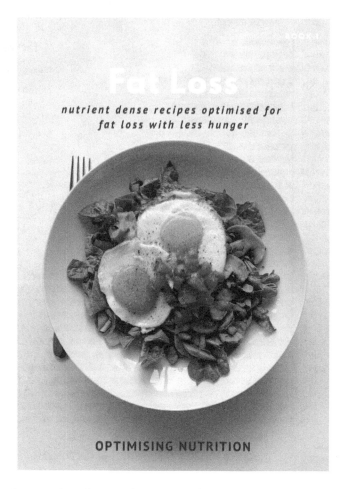

BOOK 1

Fat Loss

nutrient dense recipes optimised for
fat loss with less hunger

OPTIMISING NUTRITION

The <u>fat loss recipes</u> have a better nutrient density score and even more protein. They will enable you to get plenty of the nutrients you require to thrive, even if you are eating fewer calories overall. They are still low-carb (with only 12% net carbs) but are also lower in dietary fat to allow the fat to come from your body.

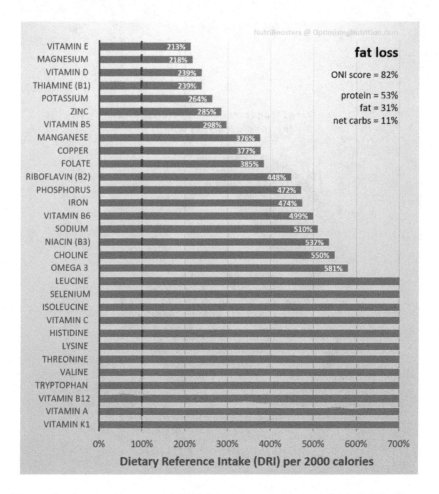

These fat-loss recipes are ideal for anyone eager to lose body fat. As we can see from the table below, it would be challenging to overeat with half the energy coming from protein. However, even with a 40% energy deficit, you would be getting plenty of protein to support lean mass retention in a deficit, while dietary carbohydrates would be low. When we combine the fat in the diet and the fat from your body, the total percentage of energy coming from fat would still be high.

energy deficit	diet (cals)	dietary fat (cals)	body fat (cals)	total fat (%)	net carb (g)	protein (g/kg LBM)
0%	2000	580	0	29%	70	4.7
10%	1800	522	200	36%	63	4.3
20%	1600	464	400	43%	56	3.8
30%	1400	406	600	50%	49	3.3
40%	1200	348	800	57%	42	2.8
50%	1000	290	1000	65%	35	2.4

High Protein:Energy Ratio

Finally, we have the high protein:energy ratio cookbook created in honour of Optimising Nutrition advisor Dr Ted Naiman for super-aggressive fat loss.

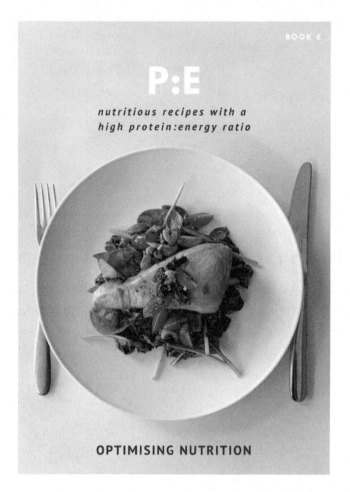

These recipes have an extremely high-protein percentage (58%) while being relatively low in both fat and carbohydrates. These will be ideal for aggressive fat loss over a short period (e.g., a bodybuilder trying to lean out for a show or someone who has a lot of body fat to lose in a hurry).

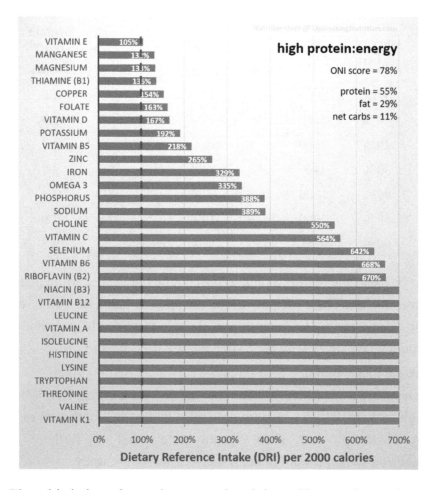

VITAMIN E — 105%
MANGANESE — 131%
MAGNESIUM — 133%
THIAMINE (B1) — 135%
COPPER — 154%
FOLATE — 163%
VITAMIN D — 167%
POTASSIUM — 192%
VITAMIN B5 — 218%
ZINC — 265%
IRON — 329%
OMEGA 3 — 335%
PHOSPHORUS — 388%
SODIUM — 389%
CHOLINE — 550%
VITAMIN C — 564%
SELENIUM — 642%
VITAMIN B6 — 668%
RIBOFLAVIN (B2) — 670%

high protein:energy

ONI score = 78%

protein = 55%
fat = 29%
net carbs = 11%

Dietary Reference Intake (DRI) per 2000 calories

The table below shows the energy breakdown if you only ate these recipes. The extremely high-protein content would make it very hard to eat enough of these meals to maintain your weight.

You could maintain a 50% energy deficit or more and still get more than enough protein to maintain lean muscle mass. Even with such high intakes of dietary protein, this may still result in endogenous ketosis (i.e., with high levels of fat coming from your body).

energy deficit	diet (cals)	dietary fat (cals)	body fat (cals)	total fat (%)	net carb (g)	protein (g/kg LBM)
0%	2000	440	0	22%	50	5.6
10%	1800	396	200	30%	45	5.1
20%	1600	352	400	38%	40	4.5
30%	1400	308	600	45%	35	3.9
40%	1200	264	800	53%	30	3.4
50%	1000	220	1000	61%	25	2.8
60%	800	176	1200	69%	20	2.3

To be clear, the high P:E recipes will not be the ideal starting place for everyone. These recipes will be the most satiating on a calorie-for-calorie basis. However, if you ate only these foods, your body would be craving easily accessible energy from fat and carbs.

So, the ideal approach is to progressively increase the protein percentage from where you are now rather than jumping from a high-fat keto diet or a modern processed diet (which both tend to provide less protein). Then, you only need to dial it up further once you stall and want to continue your fat loss journey.

Macros vs Nutrient Density

So, what are the implications for micronutrients if we simply focus on nutrient density and satiety tailored to your goal? To help us understand this, I have included some charts from the analysis of our series NutriBooster Recipe Books.

Carbohydrates

The following chart shows the relationship between non-fibre carbohydrates and nutrient density based on our analysis of the Optimiser data. There seems to be a sweet spot between 10 and 20% non-fibre carbohydrates that aligns with higher nutrient density scores.

Because nutrient-dense food has minimal amounts of processed carbs, we tend to get a reasonably low-carbohydrate outcome when we prioritise nutrients. So, while reducing carbs to stabilise your blood sugars is wise, pushing carbohydrates super-low can limit foods that can provide us with harder to find nutrients.

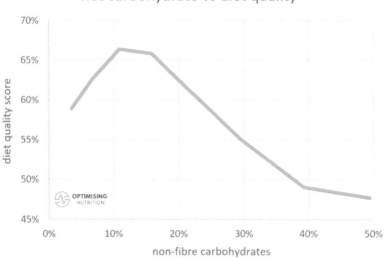

Protein

The chart below shows protein vs optimal nutrient score. The trend line shows that we get a maximum nutrient density at around 50% protein. This is a common finding from all our analysis. A higher protein percentage (up to 50%) aligns with greater nutrient density and satiety.

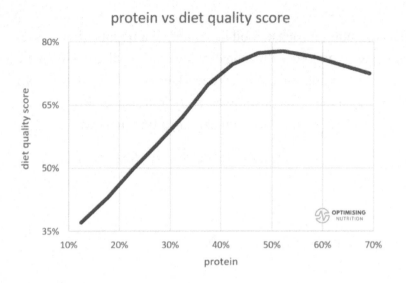

Fat

The following chart shows the percentage of fat vs <u>nutrient density</u>. While fat is an excellent source of energy that often comes packaged with protein, and there is no need to fear nutrient-dense foods that contain more fat, higher fat intake does not typically align with higher nutrient density.

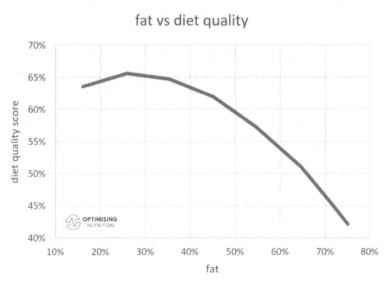

While the therapeutic keto and nutritional keto recipes may help you produce (exogenous) ketosis from the fat you are eating, they are unlikely to help you achieve endogenous ketosis as you burn your body fat.

If you want to lose fat from your body, you should look to progressively dial back both the fat and carbs in your diet while prioritising nutrient density.

Summary

Thinking simply in terms of fat or carbs being 'good' versus 'bad' is overly simplistic. Our modern food system is full of nutrient-poor processed foods that contain a mixture of fat and carbs. Once we avoid these, we get a massive improvement in nutrient density and satiety.

If you want to level up from there, you should prioritise nutrient density while tailoring the dietary fat and carbs based on whether you:

- require more energy or exogenous ketosis from the fat in your diet, or
- want to lose body fat and achieve endogenous ketosis and the many health benefits that accompany it.

Keto Lie #7: Fasting for Longer is Better

After reading this far, it may not be a surprise that I also got into the fasting craze when it was booming in Ketoland. The chart below shows my blood glucose and ketones from a seven-day fast where my blood sugars dropped, and my ketones rose to levels that my meter couldn't read.

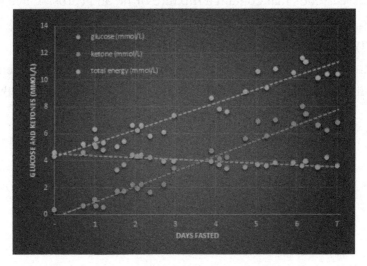

But even though I was regularly doing multi-day fasts, I still wasn't getting the results I wanted. It seemed I was gaining weight over time rather than losing. It seems I wasn't alone.

Many people fast for days at a time but are unable to lose the weight they want. It seems that losing and gaining the same few pounds is a common side effect of extended fasting.

What do you see as the biggest problems/challenges with popular fasting culture/protocols?

☐ Added by you
losing and regaining the same few lbs/kg over and over
1,291 votes

☐ Added by you
lack of emphasis on good nutrition when eating
605 votes

☐ Added by Evdoxia Renta
no weight loss despite fasting & LC routine
499 votes

☐ Added by you
no personalisation to your routine
415 votes

☐ Added by you
no quantification to ensure you are moving forward
266 votes

☐ Added by Richard Lloyd
How do you manage the after fast program to ensure post fast binging is not the probable outcome of the fast...?
229 votes

☐ Added by you
inadequate protein to prevent loss of lean mass
223 votes

☐ Added by Emma Vickers
sticking to it while hungry
153 votes

☐ Added by you
loss of healthy appetite signals
141 votes

☐ Added by Stacy Balkon Loew
What to do when it seems to stop working and tweaks aren't working
141 votes

Mark, one of our <u>Data-Driven Fasting Challenge</u> participants, observed that, although he had been doing extended fasts, his weight had simply been yo-yo-ing up and down over time.

 Mark Hannigan ▶ DDF 30-Day Challenge (25 July to 23 August 2020)
2 Aug ·

Interesting visual of my body weight in the past few months.

Each dip is an extended fast, then of course I quickly regain the weight because I wasn't thinking about what I was refeeding with and ended up binging on cheese, pork crackling and 90% chocolate 🧍 😵

The red arrow shows the start of DDF challenge 😍 😆

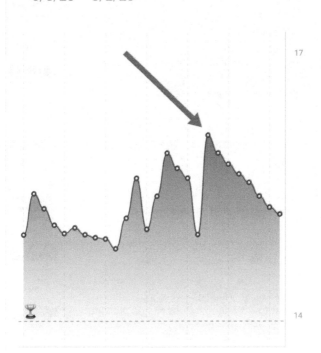

What is Fasting?

Simply put, 'fasting' is *intentionally* refraining from eating.

Jesus fasted for 40 days and 40 nights (Matthew 4:2), and Muslims do not eat during daylight hours for the month of Ramadan. However, the duration of 'fasting' can be much shorter than these commonly cited examples.

Many of us these days are accustomed to eating almost continually from soon after we wake, until just before going to bed, so an hour or two without food could be considered a fast (i.e., intentionally not eating).

Energy toxicity (not insulin toxicity) is the root cause of the majority of our modern diseases. Hence, fasting has many benefits. But rather than thinking longer is necessarily better, you need to think in terms of the *minimum effective dose* of fasting while still getting the nutrients you need when you eat.

How Long is Too Long?

While you *can* go for weeks without food, it may not be optimal for your long-term progress towards your health goals. For the many people who eat all day, a couple of hours may feel 'extended'.

There is nothing wrong with going 24 or 36 hours without food so long as you are making good choices when you refeed to ensure you are getting the nutrients you need over the longer term and don't have a history of binge eating.

However, if you are not able to control food quality or quantity when you refeed, you are unlikely to be making sustainable long-term improvements and it might be better to try shorter, but more regular fasts in the future.

Do I Need Extended Fasting or Autophagy?

Autophagy is your body's process for cleaning house and purging all the damaged cells and old protein. Autophagy literally means 'to self-eat'.

For the most part, this is a desirable thing that happens when we have less energy available from our diet. Your body starts to feed on itself, cleaning out the bits it doesn't need. Periods of low-energy availability allows our bodies to repair and purge. It's in our DNA to keep what we need, which allows us to survive and procreate another day when more food is available.

It's easy to fall into the trap of thinking that, because a little is good, more is better. We like to fit in and tend to compare ourselves with other people.

- My ketones are higher than yours.
- My blood sugar is lower than yours.
- I eat less carbs than you.
- My fast was longer than yours.

But extremes are not necessarily better, including when it comes to fasting. While there *may* be benefits of extended fasting, there are also downsides.

You may have seen images like the one below that suggest that there is something magical about fasting for a certain length of time. However, the reality is, there is no data on autophagy in humans.

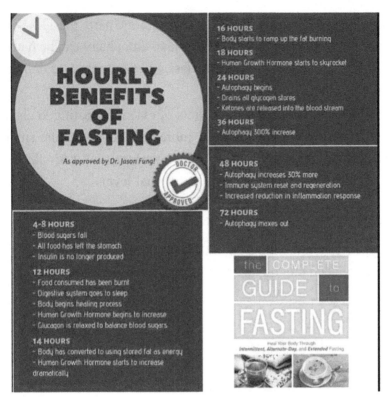

HOURLY BENEFITS OF FASTING

As approved by Dr. Jason Fung!

DOCTOR APPROVED

4-8 HOURS
- Blood sugars fall
- All food has left the stomach
- Insulin is no longer produced

12 HOURS
- Food consumed has been burnt
- Digestive system goes to sleep
- Body begins healing process
- Human Growth Hormone begins to increase
- Glucagon is relaxed to balance blood sugars

14 HOURS
- Body has converted to using stored fat as energy
- Human Growth Hormone starts to increase dramatically

16 HOURS
- Body starts to ramp up the fat burning

18 HOURS
- Human Growth Hormone starts to skyrocket

24 HOURS
- Autophagy begins
- Drains all glycogen stores
- Ketones are released into the blood stream

36 HOURS
- Autophagy 300% increase

48 HOURS
- Autophagy increases 30% more
- Immune system reset and regeneration
- Increased reduction in inflammation response

72 HOURS
- Autophagy maxes out

the COMPLETE GUIDE to FASTING

Heal Your Body Through
Intermittent, Alternate-Day, and *Extended* Fasting

Even the smartest *length* of fasting is required to achieve benefits or the minimum effective dose of fasting to achieve meaningful results. Do you need 24 hours, 36 hours, three days, seven days or maybe 14 days to get the full benefits of autophagy?

Unfortunately, studies on yeast and worms in a Petri dish aren't particularly relevant to humans living in the real world who also need to be robust and resilient to survive into old age. Italian biologist Valter Longo has shown that cycles of 48-hour fasting produce benefits in mice. But mice aren't tiny humans. One day for a mouse is equivalent to 40 human days. So, the equivalent of a 48-hour fast in a mouse (i.e., 80 days) could kill many humans.

While people often refer to Angus Barbieri, who fasted for 382 days and came out thin and healthy, they don't talk about the 10 young men in their 20s who died after not eating for between 46 and 71 days in the 1981 Irish Hunger Strike.

Autophagy occurs to some extent all the time, particularly when we are not overfed. However, too much autophagy can be harmful if you lose precious lean muscle mass when you fast and don't get enough protein when you eat.

So, rather than trusting in long stints of extended fasting to ensure you achieve autophagy, it's likely more ideal to get regular small episodes of autophagy as your critical markers (i.e., body fat, blood sugars, insulin, etc.) move towards optimal levels.

The Problem with Extended Fasting

Sadly, extended fasting does little to teach you to eat well and may lead to reduced diet quality and subsequently fat gain and muscle loss.

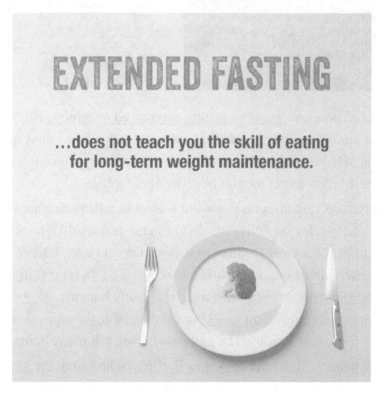

EXTENDED FASTING

...does not teach you the skill of eating for long-term weight maintenance.

You may have superpowers of self-restraint when you refeed, but most people tend to gravitate to energy-dense, nutrient-poor foods.

This means you may not get the protein and other nutrients you require in the fullness of time.

If you find yourself reaching for the peanut butter, nuts, cream or pizza after fasting, chances are you'll do better if you are a little less ambitious with your fasting duration next time.

What We Do Know About Fasting

The good news is that most of the benefits of extended fasting can be achieved by dialling in your daily meal routine (with nutrient-dense food when you do eat) to ensure a long-term energy deficit that leads to more optimal body composition.

Regular bursts of fasting, followed by nutrient dense refeeding, are much more likely to be beneficial than a few multi-day fasts followed by energy-dense, nutrient-poor binging (which can be exacerbated by a belief that fat is a free food because it will keep your insulin levels low).

While there is plenty of talk about the benefits of fasting for autophagy, cancer and Alzheimer's, there is very little data in humans to validate the theoretical benefits. What we do know is that all of these conditions are vastly improved by achieving and maintaining more optimal body composition.

As shown in the chart below, the relative risk of a range of cancers increases with increasing BMI (according to the *Quantitative association between body mass index and the risk of cancer: A global Meta-analysis of prospective cohort studies: Obesity and cancer risk*).

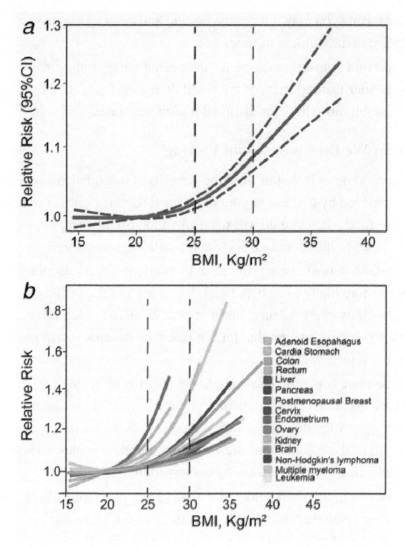

Our overall mortality risk increases with a higher BMI (chart from
*Waist-to-height Ratio Is More Predictive of Years of Life Lost
Than Body Mass Index*).

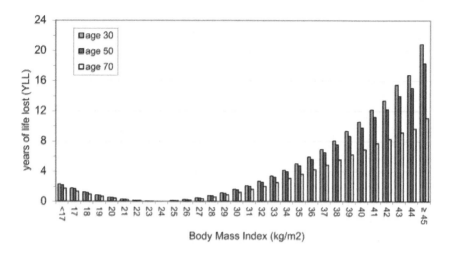

Body Mass Index (kg/m2)

Many people are concerned about insulin, mTOR and IGF-1 and hence avoid protein and fast for days or weeks, hoping to maximise autophagy and minimise these hormones. However, these things are all correlated with energy toxicity. As you bring your body fat levels down to more optimal levels, all these other things will fall into line.

To age well, as well as not be overfat, you also want to be as robust and resilient as you can be. We cannot apply theories from worms and yeast to free-living humans who need to be as strong as they can be as they age to maximise immunity, cognitive function and reduce the risk they will fall and break a hip and then never make it out of the hospital system.

J Clin Endocrinol Metab, September 2011, 96(9):2912–2920

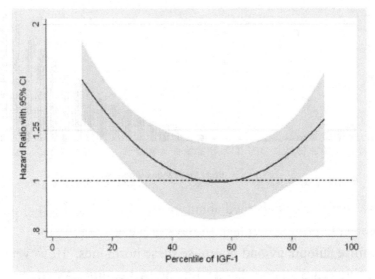

FIG. 2. Predicted HR for the association between IGF-I and all-cause mortality.

Progressive Overload for Your Metabolism

When you work out in the gym, you get progressively stronger and can lift heavier weights through 'progressive overload'. If you go all out on the first day in the gym lifting the heaviest weights you possibly can, you will be overly sore and will not return to the gym for another session for days, if ever. You are also likely to be super hungry and eat everything and anything you can to recover, thinking you've 'earned it'.

It's much more effective to build up slowly, lifting weights that stress your system a little, but that don't take you too long to recover from. You can then return to the gym on a regular basis and make progress over the long term.

Similarly, when you fast, it's much better to push your metabolism a little, but not too much that you break, so you can make consistent progress over the long term.

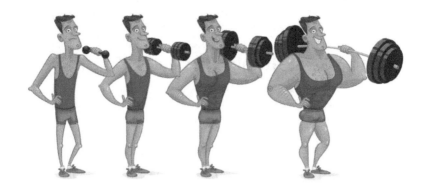

How to Optimise Your Fasting Routine to Achieve Your Goals

Many people wonder, 'How many *days* should I fast for?' However, what you really need to know is, 'How can I optimise my normal eating to ensure I am moving towards a more optimal body composition and staying below my Personal Fat Threshold?'

Keto Lie #8: Insulin Toxicity is Enemy #1.

Over the past few years, people in the fasting/low-carb/keto communities have been told that:

- insulin toxicity is the root cause of the majority of our western diseases,
- insulin is public enemy No. 1, and
- reversing 'insulin toxicity' is the key to weight loss and health.

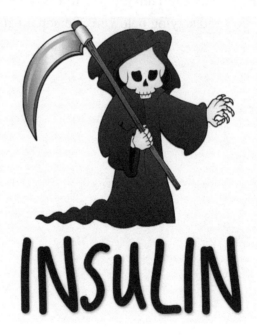

Is Fat a 'Free Food' Because #Insulin?

However, the problem with thinking in terms of 'insulin toxicity' comes when we add the belief that carbohydrates and protein will raise insulin (i.e. the *Carbohydrate Insulin Hypothesis of Obesity*) and hence dietary fat is practically a free food.

The reality is we don't have a lot of data about our insulin response to the food we eat. As shown in the example below, the data we do have (from the Food Insulin Index testing) only measures the short-term insulin response to foods *over the first two hours*.

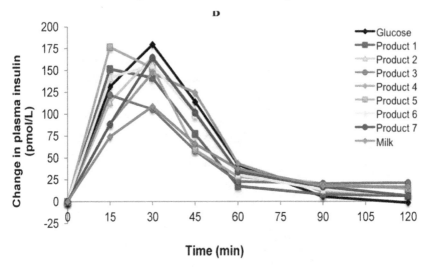

Many people extrapolate this data from the measurements we have over two hours and assume fat has no insulin response and hence they can eat almost unlimited dietary fat and t that fat is effectively a 'free food'.

While glucose will raise your insulin levels quickly, foods that contain fat and carbs together (like milk, shown by the aqua line in the chart above) will have a smaller initial impact, but insulin will stay elevated after two hours.

While we don't know that much about the long-term insulin effect of high-fat foods, it appears they also will keep our insulin levels higher over the longer term. And because fat is stored more efficiently, you don't need as much insulin to hold it in storage on your butt and belly.

It's Not Insulin Toxicity, but Energy Toxicity

Once we understand that insulin just holds our stored energy back while we use up the energy coming in from our diet, we realise that ALL food will increase insulin, to some degree, over the long term. The fundamental problem is not insulin toxicity but rather energy toxicity.

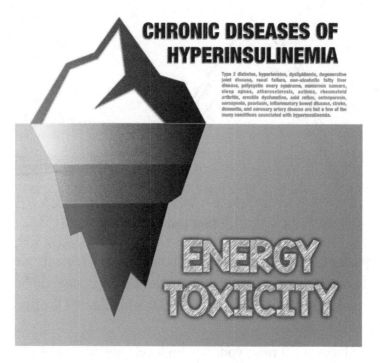

It's the excess energy that leads to increased insulin levels. Hence, the solution to decrease insulin levels is to:

- modify our food choices to achieve healthy (but not necessarily flatline) blood sugar levels, and
- reduce the amount of stored energy that requires insulin to hold in storage.

What is Diabetes?

Fundamentally, diabetes is a condition of insulin insufficiency.

- The pancreas of someone with Type 1 Diabetes cannot produce enough insulin to maintain stable blood sugars. There is often an initial 'honeymoon period' where their pancreas still produces some insulin, but in time, most people with Type 1 Diabetes produce no insulin at all. Hence, they need to take injected insulin to have enough insulin to achieve stable blood sugars.
- People with Type 2 Diabetes can produce plenty of insulin. However, because they have so much energy to hold in storage, their pancreas cannot keep up (insulin production is insufficient), and they see some of their stored energy overflows into their bloodstream.

Net Carbs vs Total Carbs vs Processed Carbs?

One of the common debates in low-carb and keto circles is whether they should be worrying about net carbs, total carbs or processed carbs to manage blood sugars, ketones, and insulin.

Processed carbs

It's often more helpful to talk about avoiding *processed* carbs. For most people, this is adequate. If you are trying to avoid nutrient-poor, low satiety foods, then avoiding foods that involve refined sugars and starches is adequate.

As shown in the satiety vs nutrient density chart here, it's typically these refined carbs that are added to 'vegetable oils' that end up being 'bad carbs' that people intuitively know that they should avoid (e.g. doughnuts, cookies, croissants, etc.).

Meanwhile, there is no need for most people to avoid non-starchy vegetables. They will be hard to overeat, and you will get plenty of the harder-to-find nutrients per calorie.

Net carbs or non-fibre carbs?

"Net carbs" refers to the total carbohydrates minus the fibre in your food.

Net Carbs = Total Carbohydrates – Carbohydrates from Fibre

It's hard to overeat foods that naturally contain a lot of bulk and fibre. Fibre doesn't count towards your overall calorie intake because, for the most part, it isn't digested in your gut to provide calories or significantly raise your blood sugar.

The chart below shows how thinking about net carbs can be more effective to dial in satiety. Moving from moderate to lower total carbohydrates aligns with a 21% reduction in calories. In contrast, decreasing net carbs instead gives us a more substantial 29% reduction in calories.

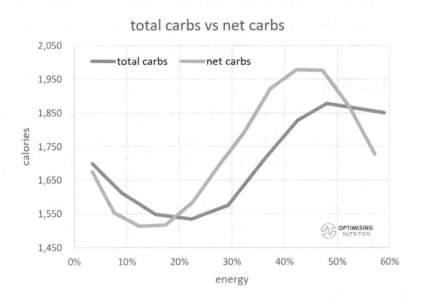

For the most part, fibre is not available to be used by your body for energy and hence will not raise blood sugars or insulin. It is fermented in the gut to feed gut bacteria or is excreted undigested. Fibre is not necessarily a goal that you need to strive to get a certain minimum amount of. However, nutrient-dense, high-satiety foods tend to contain plenty of fibre.

The problem with thinking in terms of total carbs rather than net carbs is when we have people who want to lose weight avoiding foods like lettuce, broccoli and spinach for fear they will be getting too many carbohydrates because it will kick them out of ketosis, spike their insulin and make them fat.

If you find you are insulin resistant and your blood sugars rise more than 1.6 mmol/L (or 30 mg/dL) after meals, then it can be helpful to think in terms of managing your net carbs or non-fibre carbs.

If you are working to a carbohydrate limit, we recommend most people think in terms of 'net carbs without sugar alcohols' (you can select this setting in Cronometer).

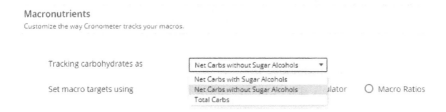

Sugar alcohols are typically contained in processed foods to make them sweeter and more palatable (hence you will likely eat more of them). Some of them will raise your blood sugars while others won't (see the glycemic index of sweeteners here).

Double Diabetes

The line between Type 1 and Type 2 Diabetes is not always clear. Some people develop what is known as 'Double Diabetes'.

For someone with Type 1 Diabetes, years of injecting large amounts of insulin that drive hunger and overeating mean they develop increased insulin resistance due to increased levels of body fat. As a result, they require more basal insulin to hold their stored energy in storage when not eating, and when they do eat, they will need more insulin for their meals. When people with Type 1 Diabetes lose weight, we see their basal insulin requirements plummet, and their insulin sensitivity improves, so they need less insulin for meals.

Conversely, someone with Type 2 Diabetes, after a number of years, may find their pancreas effectively burns out, and their beta cells are no longer able to produce as much insulin. At this point, they will need to take more and more insulin.

Sadly, two-thirds of the insulin produced today is used by people with Type 2 Diabetes, which could potentially be avoided with diet and exercise. People with Type 1 Diabetes may be taking 10 to 40 units of insulin per day, while someone with poorly controlled Type 2 Diabetes may be taking more than 200 units of insulin per day due to their extreme insulin resistance.

What's the Solution?

If we want to maximise our insulin sensitivity and lose fat from our body, it's not merely a matter of eating fewer carbs and more fat, as some people would have us believe.

Modifying our diet (i.e., reducing processed carbs) will only marginally decrease the insulin requirements in response to meals (i.e., bolus insulin).

While reducing the processed carbohydrates in your diet will help to reduce the amount of insulin required for meals, we need to keep in mind that the basal insulin (i.e., the insulin produced by our pancreas or injected to maintain stable blood sugars when we don't eat) comprises the majority of the insulin requirements across the day.

In someone consuming a typical high-carb diet, basal insulin makes up around 50% of their insulin requirements. However, for someone following a low-carb or keto diet, the basal insulin may make up <u>80 to 90% of their total daily insulin dose</u> (TDD).

To reduce insulin, we need to optimise our diet for greater <u>satiety</u>, which will lead to a reduction in stored energy, lower blood sugars, improved insulin sensitivity and reduced basal insulin. Additionally, improvements in insulin sensitivity will lead to reduced insulin requirements for food.

How to Optimise Your Diet for Fat Loss and Reduce Insulin

Stabilise Blood Sugars with Better Food Choices

In our <u>Macros Masterclass</u> and <u>Data-Driven Fasting,</u> we encourage people to monitor their blood sugar rise after meals. If blood sugar rises by more than 1.6 mmol/L (or 30 mg/dL), then it is a great idea to look to reduce the carbohydrates (i.e., net carbs or non-fibre carbs) to the point that the blood sugars stabilise to healthy, non-diabetic levels.

However, if your blood sugars are already below this threshold, there is little value in trying to stabilise your blood sugars even further, especially if this involves swapping out carbohydrates for fat. On the other hand, if you already have healthy blood sugar levels, then you can get on with prioritising nutrient density and satiety.

Prioritise Satiety and Nutrient Density

If you still have body fat to lose, the next step is to simply prioritise foods and meals that provide greater satiety and nutrient density (they typically go together). In the <u>Macros Masterclass</u>, we use <u>Nutrient Optimiser</u> to guide you to:

- ensure you are getting adequate protein to prevent loss of lean muscle mass.
- dial back non-fibre carbohydrates (if blood sugars are still elevated).

- dial back dietary fat (to allow body fat to be used); and
- prioritise foods and meals that contain more of the nutrients you are struggling to get enough of.

This process can continue until a healthy level of body fat is achieved (i.e., waist:height ratio of less than 0.5 or less than 15% body fat for men and less than 25% body fat for women). By doing this, we will reduce both basal and bolus insulin requirements and vastly improve insulin sensitivity.

For more detail, see Macronutrients [Macros Masterclass FAQ #2].

Meal Timing

In the Data-Driven Fasting Challenge, we use pre-meal blood sugars to guide meal timing to ensure an overall energy deficit is being achieved. If blood sugars are low and stable, but weight loss is not occurring, then we encourage people to increase the protein percentage of their meals by dialling back dietary fat to allow body fat to be used.

If your blood sugars are already in the healthy range and you are not injecting insulin to manage your diabetes, rather than worrying so much about your rise in blood sugars and insulin after meals, it's more beneficial to monitor your blood sugars before meals and delay/or skip them until they return to below your baseline.

Waiting for your blood sugars to return to baseline will ensure you are not over-fuelling. But, waiting a little longer until they are a little lower empowers you to validate your hunger and ensure a long-term energy deficit that will reverse energy toxicity.

How to Optimise Your Type 1 Diabetes Management

The process is similar to the process above, with the following additional considerations if you are injecting insulin.

- Monitoring blood sugar becomes important to ensure basal

insulin is titrated back to prevent low blood sugars (i.e., less than 4.0 mmol/L or 72 mg/dL). As you lose fat, you will require less basal insulin to keep your blood sugars stable when you don't eat.

- If you are using an insulin pump, you will need to increase your Insulin Sensitivity Factor (i.e., the amount by which a certain amount of insulin will lower your blood sugar). You will also need to increase your insulin-to-carb ratio as you will need less insulin for a given amount of carbohydrates.
- Finally, once your blood sugars stabilise and there is less variability, you can target a lower average blood sugar across the day to achieve an average blood glucose level similar to a metabolically healthy person. For example, if you have not experienced a blood sugar below 4.0 mmol/L or 72 mg/dL for the past week, you can target a slightly lower blood sugar for the coming week.

Keto Lie #9: Calories Don't Count

M any find low-carb or keto almost magical in the early days. As they move away from the most hyperpalatable fat+carb combo foods, they experience greater satiety, their blood sugars and insulin levels drop, and they feel great.

High-fat foods can also *feel* satiating, but this may be simply because they quickly provide you with a lot of energy. Many popular low-carb or keto foods contain plenty of bioavailable protein, so they get a great satiety response. Folks are suddenly able to manage their food intake without having to fight against their appetite.

It's no wonder that, after trying to count calories and restrict, once they switch to a low-carb diet, they start to believe that calories don't matter.

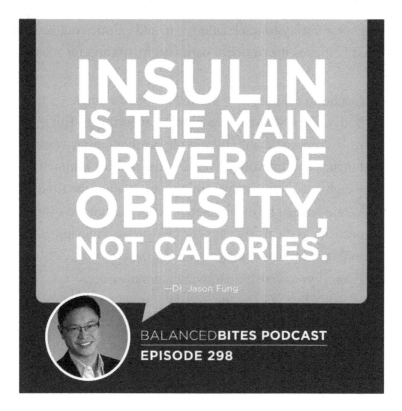

INSULIN
IS THE MAIN
DRIVER OF
OBESITY,
NOT CALORIES.

—Dr. Jason Fung

BALANCED**BITES** PODCAST
EPISODE 298

But the problem comes when they also think fat is a 'free food' and steer the ship towards more refined fat rather than whole-food protein sources, believing that it's all about keeping insulin low rather than energy balance. Unfortunately, most people don't get away with unlimited added fats like cream, butter and oil while continuing to lose body fat over the long term.

But, when keto fails, is counting calories the next logical step? And if not, what else can we do to continue our fat-loss journey?

The Problem with Counting Calories

In the end, energy balance still matters. All calories count, but only if you can accurately count all the calories going in and coming out.

However, the reality is that energy is hard for us to balance simply by counting calories with a smartphone app paired with our fitness trackers. Our ability to track calories in and calories out accurately and reliably makes it extremely hard and frustrating for most people.

- Counting calories may be fine if you're a single bodybuilder who can pre-prepare everything. But most of us live unpredictable lives with family dinners, work lunches and impromptu parties that make it impractical to weigh and measure everything we eat all of the time.
- While we can be disciplined *most* of the time, it's those occasional meals (when your calorie tracking app isn't looking) that undo all your hard work.
- Even if you were able to weigh and measure EVERYTHING you ate, the data in your app rarely matches the foods you are eating.
- Your body doesn't 'burn' the food the same way that calories are measured in a bomb calorimeter (shown below).

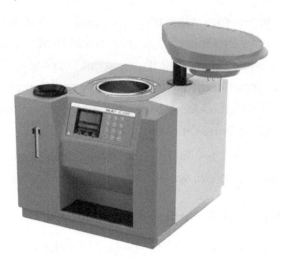

- Your calorie tracking app doesn't account for the thermic effect of food, which changes depending on the macronutrient profile of your food and the degree of processing.

- Foods that are more processed tend to be easily digested, while foods that are less processed are more likely to be digested slowly and keep us feeling fuller for longer or be excreted.

- Any calorie target from an online calculator is going to be inaccurate. Your metabolism is complex, and the number of calories you require depends on various factors, including your muscle mass, exercise, stress and sleep (not to mention pandemics and lockdowns, which restrict your movement).

- Your energy expenditure changes from day to day. If you try to maintain a fixed calorie intake, there is a serious risk that your healthy appetite signals will become dysregulated as you try to push through hunger some days and overeat on others.

- When you suddenly slash your energy intake, your body quickly adapts to survive. Your metabolic rate slows. You produce less heat. You feel less energetic, and your involuntary activity will reduce. You 'burn' fewer calories day to day than you used to.

- Any estimate of your energy expenditure that you get from your FitBit or Oura ring is only an estimate and is likely to be highly inaccurate. People who rely on these devices to estimate their calorie expenditure are more likely to gain weight because they tend to congratulate themselves and eat back the calories the app has told them they burned.

- When you count calories, your focus remains on how much you can eat rather than listening to your body's hunger signals, which tell you when you need to eat.

- Simply counting calories teaches you nothing about food quality and a sustainable eating pattern that will lead to long-term health.

Eating should be impulsive and instinctual. Your body drives your appetite to ensure you seek out the nutrients you need. However, it also means that, despite our best efforts to limit the amount we eat, our appetite usually wins out, especially if we continue to eat the same food that led us to be overfat in the first place.

So, while energy is always conserved, the factors on either side of the calories in vs calories out equation are incredibly complex and beyond our ability to manage accurately.

Calorie Tracking Can Cause You to Develop an Eating Disorder

If you've ever tried tracking your calories, you will understand that your reptilian brain doesn't like to relinquish control of your appetite to a smartphone app. As shown in the image below, your brain is divided up into three portions.

- The neocortex is the rational or thinking part of our brain. This is the logical part of your brain that makes plans to lose weight and eat less using the latest technology.
- The limbic brain is the part that feels emotions (which may not always appear logical or align with what your neocortex is thinking).
- Then we have the reptilian brain, which looks after basic survival functions like breathing, temperature control and eating.

Your Actions Are Not Your Own

Your Three Brains

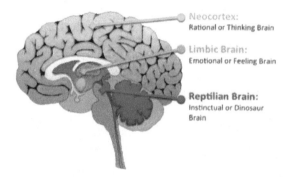

Neocortex:
Rational or Thinking Brain

Limbic Brain:
Emotional or Feeling Brain

Reptilian Brain:
Instinctual or Dinosaur
Brain

While calories in vs calories out sounds seductively simple, your reptilian instincts fight for control when awoken by the threat of starvation! It's critical to keep your 'inner lizard' fed with high-quality food, so it doesn't sense an emergency and stays asleep.

Many people become anxious when they put so much effort into tracking everything they eat and don't get the results they hoped for. Sadly, food tracking can drive an unhealthy neurosis in many people.

A 2017 study of people with a diagnosed eating disorder found that 75% of participants reported using MyFitnessPal. Disturbingly, 73% of the MyFitnessPal users said that their use of MyFitnessPal had *contributed* to their eating disorder.

Hopefully, you can see by now that simply counting calories and trying to stay under some arbitrary target using self-restraint while continuing to eat the same foods doesn't end well for most people. This is why it's essential to prioritise nutrient-dense high-satiety foods to enable you to manage your appetite.

Precision vs Accuracy in Food Tracking

While food tracking is rarely accurate and reliable, it *can* still be helpful if we understand its limitations. To help explain what I mean by this, the image below shows the difference between accuracy and reliability.

Let's consider the target in the top left (i.e., accurate and reliable). It is unlikely you're going to be perfectly *accurate* and *reliable* in your food tracking (top left target) at the same time due to the inaccuracies related to food labelling and measurement. This is what most people expect from their tracking, but it just doesn't occur in the real world.

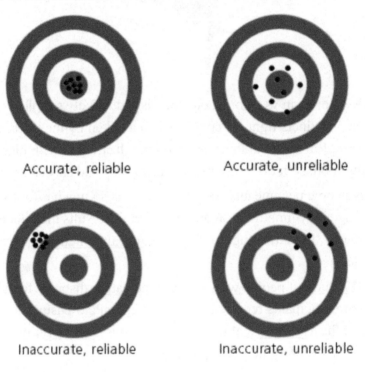

Accurate, reliable   Accurate, unreliable

Inaccurate, reliable   Inaccurate, unreliable

A bodybuilder preparing for a contest who weighs and measures everything they eat and consumes a regimented diet may be inaccurate and reliable (bottom left corner). They will be eating similar things day to day, week to week, with slight modifications to make sure they keep moving forward. Even though their estimation of calories is not *accurate*, they are *reliable*, so their food tracking data is valuable.

Most people who are tracking their food intake will be *inaccurate* and *unreliable* (bottom right target). While not as powerful, this data can still be useful so long as you can update your target macros based on your actual progress in terms of fat loss, blood sugars and retention of lean mass.

Note: Developing a regular eating routine with an appropriate level of variety is helpful to maximise sensory-specific satiety. *Constant novelty and variety will cause you to eat more, making it harder to be reliable or accurate.*

Why Managing Macros is More Useful than Tracking Calories

While trying to stay under some arbitrary calorie target is a fool's errand, it may be useful to track your macronutrients (i.e., carbs, fat and protein). Together with your biometric data (i.e., weight, body fat and blood sugars), you can use this information to ensure you continue to move towards optimal metabolic health.

- If your blood sugar regularly rises by more than 1.6 mmol/L (or 30 mg/dL) after meals, then it's likely you are eating excessive amounts of refined carbohydrates and need to adjust your carbohydrate limit.
- If you are losing excessive amounts of lean mass (i.e., muscle), then you likely need more protein.
- If you are still not losing weight, then you likely need to dial back your dietary fat intake to ensure fat is coming from your body rather than your plate or coffee mug.

For more details on our Smart Macros Algorithm, *check out the article* Why set and forget calorie targets will always fail you (and how Smart Macros Algorithm can help).

What to Do When Weight Loss Stalls

- If you have stopped making your desired progress, we recommend people try <u>Data-Driven Fasting</u>, using the blood sugar meter as a fuel gauge to be sure to achieve a negative energy balance (without counting calories). This is simple and effective for most people, with the minimum investment of time and effort and avoids the hassle of food tracking.

- For those who find their blood sugars are super stable but are still not seeing weight loss, we recommend checking their macronutrient profile by tracking in <u>Cronometer</u> for a few days. If your goal is fat loss, you can work towards a 40% protein. If your blood sugars are already stable, this can be achieved by dialling back dietary fat while focusing on nutrient-dense foods.

- If you're looking for guidance on how much protein and fat you should be eating, you can use this <u>simple macro calculator</u> as a starting point.

- If you're motivated to track your food, you can use our <u>*7-Day Nutrient Clarity Challenge*</u> to review your micronutrients and identify the foods and meals you should focus on to achieve your goal.

Keto Lie #10: Stable Blood Sugars Will Lead to Fat Loss

If there was anything I thought I knew for sure when I was an insulin-fearing keto zealot, it was that:

- the blood sugar rollercoaster is bad, and
- stable blood sugars were good.

According to the keto gurus that I was following, if you want to lose fat and optimise your metabolic health, the most important thing you could do is to eat fewer carbs to achieve flatline blood sugars and 'turn off your insulin'.

Even today, there is still plenty of confusion about the role of stable blood sugars and insulin levels in weight loss.

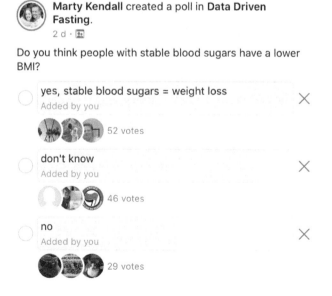

Marty Kendall created a poll in **Data Driven Fasting.**
2 d ·

Do you think people with stable blood sugars have a lower BMI?

yes, stable blood sugars = weight loss
Added by you
52 votes   ✕

don't know
Added by you
46 votes   ✕

no
Added by you
29 votes   ✕

Many people incorrectly assume that super-stable blood sugars will lead to lower insulin levels, which will automatically lead to fat loss.

Since we started Data-Driven Fasting, I have had a barrage of questions as people try to make sense of their blood sugars. Now that thousands of people have completed their baselining phase of Data-Driven Fasting, we have data demonstrating that eating a high-fat diet to stabilise your blood sugar is unlikely to help you lose weight.

Rather than worrying about your blood glucose *after* meals, your blood glucose *before* meals is a more powerful way to optimise your metabolic health. By actively managing your blood glucose levels *before* you eat (through meal timing and nutrient-focused foods and meals), you can optimise the numbers that matter when managing your metabolic health (i.e., BMI, waist-to-height ratio and waking blood sugars).

What We Know From People With Type 1 Diabetes

For someone with Type 1 Diabetes, injecting large doses of insulin to treat elevated blood sugars from modern processed food leaves them on a blood sugar rollercoaster. When their blood sugars are high, they inject more insulin to bring their blood sugars down.

A few hours later, when they find they have overshot their blood sugar target, they are ravenously hungry and will eat anything and everything in sight until they can raise their blood sugars again. A day in the life of most people living with Type 1 Diabetes looks like this. In this scenario, *injected insulin is driving their appetite and causing them to eat more.*

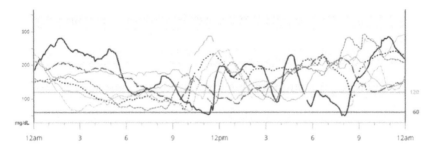

If their insulin doses are not precisely matched with the food they eat (which is nearly impossible with synthetic, injected insulin combined with synthetic, processed food), they end up overeating *because* of the insulin they are injecting.

Living with rollercoaster blood sugars sucks – appetite, mood or energy levels are in the toilet!

How Insulin Really Works

While we often think of insulin as the hormone that jams energy *into* our cells, it's not the whole story.

We all have about 5 grams of glucose (about a teaspoon or 20 calories worth) buzzing around in our bloodstream at any one time. It doesn't take long to use this up once we turn off the flow of energy into our bloodstream.

If you could turn off the release of energy from your liver completely, you would run out of glucose in about 15 minutes.

Insulin is secreted by the pancreas that turns off the flow of stored energy into your bloodstream (from your liver and adipose tissue) until you burn up the energy in your blood from that last meal.

So, rather than thinking of insulin as an anabolic hormone (i.e. it helps things to grow), it's much more helpful to focus on its function as an anti-catabolic hormone (i.e. it stops us from breaking down and disintegrating).

As per Dr Bernstein's *Law of Small Numbers*, once people with Type 1 Diabetes reduce the significant inputs of processed carbohydrates that require large doses of insulin, they can stabilise their blood sugars and insulin requirements.

Smaller inputs of carbs and insulin lead to smaller errors that are easier to correct throughout the day. When they are no longer injecting massive amounts of insulin to treat the blood sugar rollercoaster, their appetite stabilises, and they tend to achieve healthy body fat levels.

If you are part of the one in 8000 people with Type 1 Diabetes whose pancreas doesn't work, stabilising your blood sugars and insulin by manipulating your diet should be your highest priority.

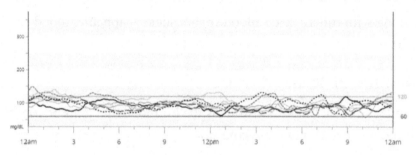

The Difference Between People with Type 1 Diabetes and Everyone Else!

If you are part of the 99.5% of the population that is fortunate enough to have a functioning pancreas, EVERYTHING is different.

You cannot turn off your insulin pump or stop injecting insulin. No matter what we'd *like* to believe, it just doesn't work like that.

Your pancreas will *always* produce just enough insulin (no more, no less) to hold your body fat in storage until you have used up the extra energy from the food coming in from your mouth. Then, when you stop eating, insulin levels lower and your stored energy is allowed to be released for use.

If you have Type 2 Diabetes and eat a diet of heavily processed carbs and fat (e.g., modern processed junk food), your blood sugars will shoot up after eating and take a long time to come back down.

But What if I'm 'Insulin Resistant'?

'Insulin resistance' is a term that is used a lot in low-carb and keto circles. But why we become insulin resistant and how to reverse it is not yet commonly understood. Many people think they are obese because they are insulin resistant. But the reverse is true. They are insulin resistant because they are obese.

When your fat cells (which make up your adipose tissue) fill up (like a sponge or a balloon), it becomes harder to force more energy into them. As a result, your pancreas must raise insulin levels more and more to enable your body to continue to store excess energy. Because we need more and more insulin to do the job, the fat cells appear to have become resistant to the effects of insulin, and thus, we say we have become insulin resistant.

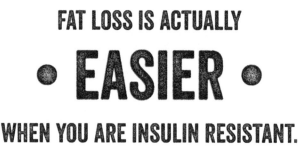

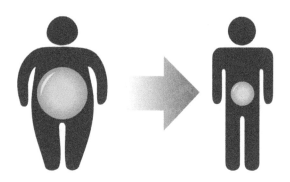

Many people develop a victim mentality (I was one of them), believing that they are insulin resistant. They blame their obesity on their insulin resistance (not the other way around). They think being insulin resistant makes it harder for them to lose weight, but the reverse is true.

This chart shows the weight loss in our first Macros Masterclass for people who identified themselves as insulin resistant vs insulin sensitive. It was interesting to see that people who identified themselves as insulin resistant lost weight at a similar rate as everybody else. In the end, it was actually the people who believed they were insulin resistant who lost slightly more weight.

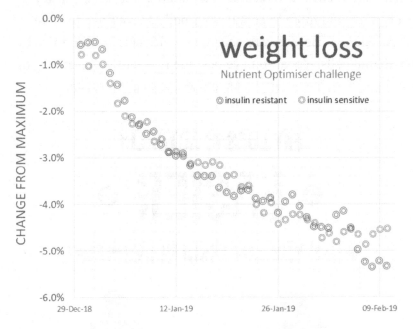

When you are lean and insulin sensitive, your body is eager to store energy and grow. However, once you become insulin resistant, your body is only too willing to offload the excess energy as soon as you stop jamming in low-satiety, nutrient-poor processed foods.

The chart below shows the difference between diabetic and healthy blood sugar levels (i.e., higher and with bigger swings). Foods that are a combination of fat+carb together enable your body to fill both fuel tanks at the same time. Because your fat stores are already full, the extra energy is not easily absorbed by your liver and body fat, so it overflows into your bloodstream.

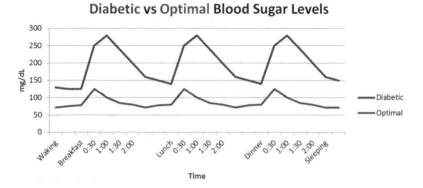

You can't blame getting fat on insulin. It's the nutrient-poor foods with carbs and fat (together with low protein) that cause you to overeat and gain fat. The increase in insulin is simply the consequence of storing more energy on your body.

Once you're carrying extra body fat, you require lots of extra insulin to hold it in. Understanding the cause-and-effect relationship is critical to designing the correct dietary solution.

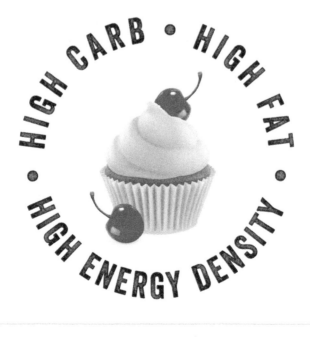

It's not that stable blood sugars are a bad thing. But simply switching carbs for fat to achieve stable blood sugars is nothing more than symptom management. It won't make you lean and metabolically healthy and may even make things worse!

Show Me the Science!

Since launching the <u>Data-Driven Fasting</u>, we have been bombarded with questions about blood sugars and insulin as people test their blood sugars and try to make sense of the data they see.

- Why do my blood sugars rise when I don't eat?
- How much should my blood sugars rise after I eat?
- My blood sugars are flatline? Why am I not losing fat?

With data from hundreds of people, I have been able to understand if there is really a relationship between more stable blood sugars and fat loss.

Flatline Blood Sugar Envy... We're Still Chasing the Wrong Numbers

Many people believe that maintaining stable blood glucose levels is the highest priority and will lead to weight loss.

I'm seeing more and more people (who don't have Type 1 Diabetes) walking around with (expensive and sometimes painful) continuous glucose monitors (CGMs) eating more fat and less protein and carbs to make sure they maintain flatline blood sugars. They proudly post their flatline blood sugars on Facebook and Instagram.

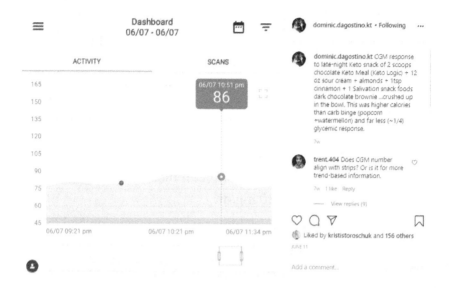

How Much Should My Blood Sugars Rise After a Meal?

To help us understand how much our blood sugar should rise after a meal, the table below shows the generally accepted limits for blood glucose.

	Fasting		After meal		Glucose rise	
	mg/dL	mmol/L	mg/dL	mmol/L	mg/dL	mmol/L
Normal	< 100	< 5.6	< 140	< 7.8	< 40	< 2.2
Pre-diabetic	100 – 126	5.6 - 7.0	140 - 200	7.8 - 11.1	40 - 74	2.2 - 4.1
Type 2 Diabetes	> 126	> 7.0	> 200	> 11.1	> 75	> 4.1

If your blood sugars after meals are elevated above 7.8 mmol/L (140 mg/dL), then you have prediabetes or diabetes and need to work to reduce your post-meal blood glucose by reducing refined carbohydrates and/or medications to reduce blood sugars. This maximum peak usually occurs within an hour or two after you eat, depending on the type of food.

A rise in glucose from 5.6 mmol/L to 7.8 mmol/L (100 mg/dL to

140 mg/dL) would be accepted as normal and healthy. If your blood sugars rise by less than 2.6 mmol/L or 40 mg/dL, then it's highly likely you have a fully functioning pancreas, and you would benefit by focusing on your blood sugars *before* you eat (not after) if you have more weight to lose.

In the Macros Masterclass and Data-Driven Fasting, we set even tighter limits than this. We recommend that people reduce the amount of processed carbs in their diet if their blood sugars rise by more than 1.6 mmol/L or 30 mg/dL.

Once your blood sugars are stable, you should move on and focus on nutrient density, satiety and your blood sugars *before* meals rather than continuing to micromanage the fluctuations in your blood sugars after you eat in the mistaken belief that this will help. Interestingly, the average rise for people following Data-Driven Fasting is only 10 mg/dL or 0.5 mmol/L, which is not much. It seems people who are fans of fasting (and typically following a low-carb or keto style diet) already have *extremely* stable blood sugars! However, many of them still have a lot of fat to lose.

Stable Blood Glucose Does Not Equal Fat Loss!

The charts from the data from people using Data-Driven Fasting below show there is no correlation between someone's waist:height ratio or BMI and their blood sugar after they eat.

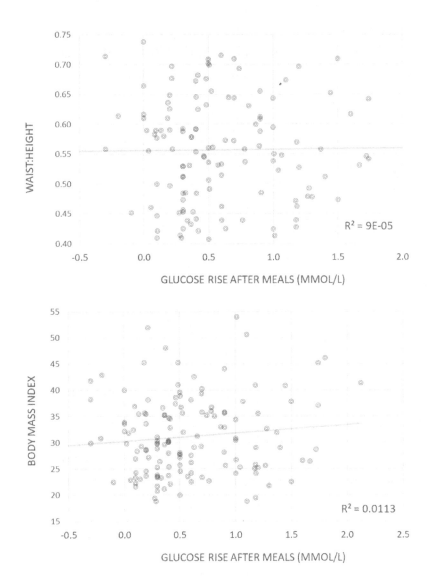

There is also no correlation between the amount your blood glucose rises after you eat and your waking blood glucose (another critical marker of metabolic health). Although it's good to have stable blood sugars in the healthy range, flatline is not better, especially if you had to consume a low <u>satiety</u>, high-fat, nutrient-poor diet to get it!

Although stable and lower blood glucose levels are a positive marker of good metabolic health, merely treating the symptom (i.e., elevated blood sugar) rather than addressing the cause (i.e., energy toxicity and excess body fat) doesn't help.

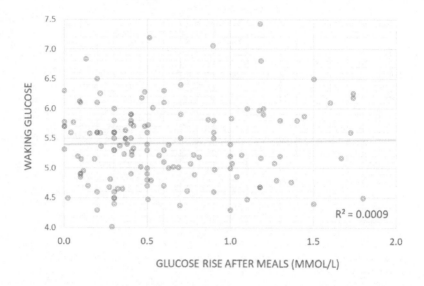

Unfortunately, many people who believe fat is a 'free food' because it does not raise insulin significantly in the short term after eating end up overeating fat in a misguided effort to maintain stable blood sugar levels. Before long, this can quickly lead to fat gain. Excessive levels of stored energy on the body lead to high insulin levels across the day to hold the fat in storage.

Blood Glucose Variability

When we look at blood glucose variability (i.e., standard deviation/average glucose), we see there is also a negligible correlation between stable blood sugars and a better waist:height ratio, BMI or waking blood sugars.

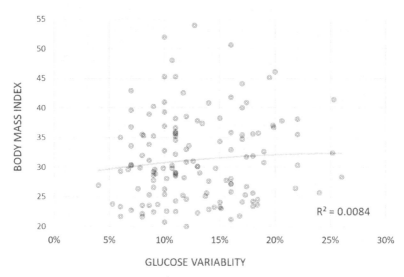

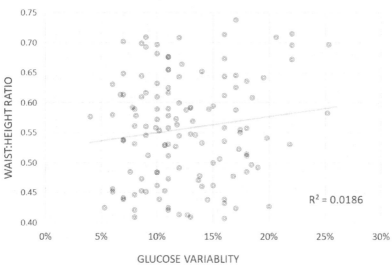

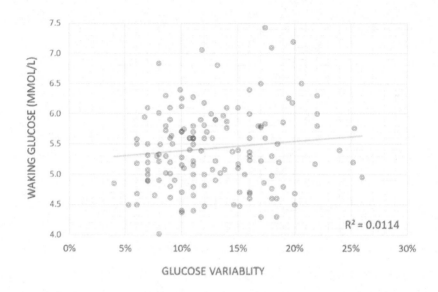

Many people combine fasting with a high-fat keto diet to achieve stable blood sugars in the hope of weight loss and/or improved health. But sadly, despite their herculean feats of self-deprivation, they just continue to gain weight due to a low-satiety, nutrient-poor diet that leaves them craving and eating more when they break their fast.

Actively avoiding insulin and rises in blood sugar levels using a high-fat diet tends to lead to poorer satiety, greater energy intake and obesity. In time, these people end up with *higher* insulin levels across the day because they are carrying more body fat, which requires more insulin to hold in storage.

At this point, you may be thinking that measuring blood sugar is completely useless. This is not what I'm saying. Wild swings in blood sugar outside the normal healthy range are not ideal. But rather than simply being intolerant to carbohydrates, the reality is, a large rise in blood glucose after you eat is likely due to fuel (from both fat and glucose) backing up in your system.

A low-carb or keto diet does help to stabilise the swings in blood glucose. However, managing the symptom of diabetes by trying to achieve minimal blood sugar variation by avoiding all carbs and even protein does not address the root cause and may even make things worse.

Pre-Meal Trigger

Because glucose is such a volatile fuel and effectively floats on top of all the fat in your body, measuring your blood sugar when you wake or BEFORE YOU EAT is an excellent way to ensure you are not chronically over-fuelling (from either fat or carbs).

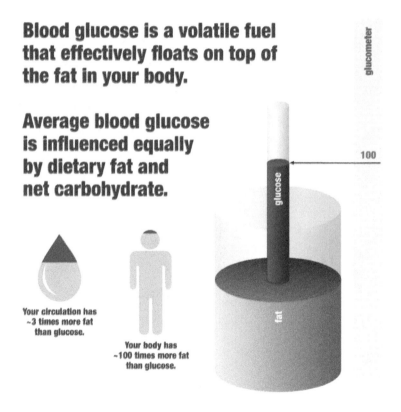

Blood glucose is a volatile fuel that effectively floats on top of the fat in your body.

Average blood glucose is influenced equally by dietary fat and net carbohydrate.

Your circulation has ~3 times more fat than glucose.

Your body has ~100 times more fat than glucose.

As shown in the charts below, we see a much better correlation between a pre-meal blood glucose trigger and waist:height ratio and waking glucose. Rather than worrying so much about your blood sugars *after* you eat, it seems that people who have lower blood glucose *before they eat* tend to have much better metabolic health.

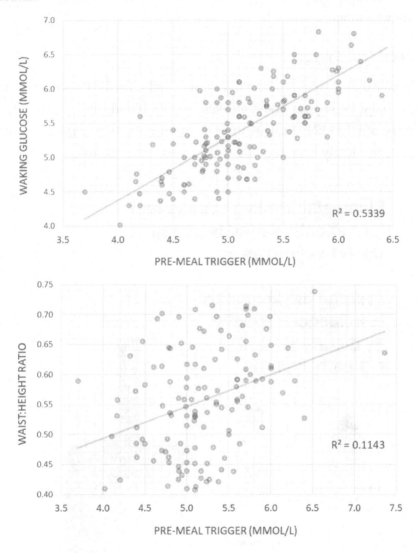

There is some variability across individuals due to different Personal Fat Thresholds. However, when we look at this on a person-by-person basis as they progressively lower their premeal blood sugars (e.g. Jane's data below), we see that a lower pre-meal blood glucose trigger before you eat aligns nicely with weight and body fat levels.

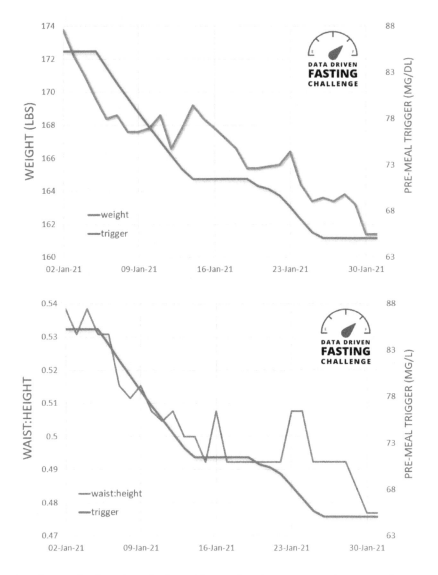

As shown in the chart below (from the *Association between fasting glucose and all-cause mortality* study), your waking glucose is one of the most powerful indicators of metabolic health and your risk of *dying from any cause*.

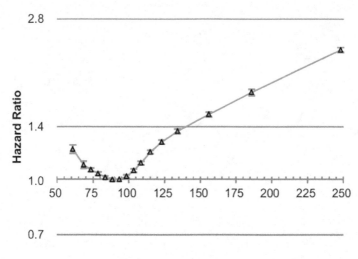

Fasting Serum Glucose (mg/dL)

Pre-meal blood glucose trigger strongly correlates with your waking blood glucose. Rather than worrying about the rise in blood glucose *after* you eat, managing your blood glucose *before* you eat is much more useful if you want to lose fat and gain health!

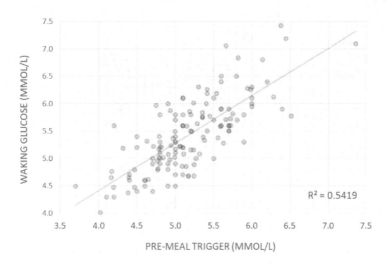

To optimise body composition, you need to measure and manage the things that matter. Your blood sugar before meals is an extremely useful thing to measure, and you can manage it by simply optimising your meal timing/intermittent fasting routine to ensure it continues to decrease.

Doesn't WHAT I Eat Matter Too?

WHAT you eat is arguably more important than WHEN you eat. Data-Driven Fasting simply empowers you to optimise your food timing to ensure a negative energy balance.

- While high-fat foods and meals will keep your blood sugars stable, they also provide a lot of energy, along with lower satiety. Although your blood sugars and insulin levels may be stable, your body won't need to draw down on your body fat until it burns up all the energy from that fat bomb or buttered coffee.
- Meals with more fast-digesting, non-fibre carbohydrates will raise your blood sugars quickly, but they will likely return to below baseline more quickly as well.
- Foods that contain both fat and carbs together (which are typically also low in protein) will fill your fat and glucose fuel tanks at the same time and allow you to eat more, and keep your blood sugars elevated for longer.
- Foods with a higher percentage of protein and a greater nutrient density are harder to overeat and won't raise your blood sugars significantly (in fact, they may reduce them). Your blood glucose will return to below target more quickly.

Avoiding Blood Sugar Spikes is Only the First Step

In our Macros Masterclass, we guide people to reduce their carbohydrates if their blood sugars rise more than 30 mg/dL or 1.6 mmol/L after meals. But once they achieve this, there is no benefit in avoiding nutrient-dense foods that may contain some carbohydrates.

As they fill in their nutrient gaps (by chasing the nutrients they are currently struggling to get enough of, as demonstrated in the nutrient fingerprint chart below) with more nutrient-dense foods, they eliminate all the problematic nutrient-poor processed carbs anyway.

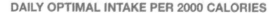

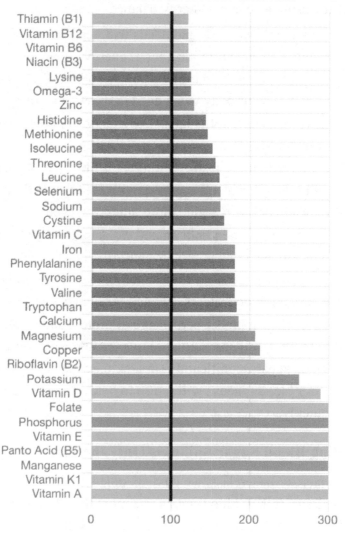

DAILY OPTIMAL INTAKE PER 2000 CALORIES

Optimal Nutrition Score for your food log is 100%.

In our Data-Driven Fasting Challenge, we guide people to reduce
or eliminate foods and meals that are causing their blood glucose
to rise more than 30 mg/dL or 1.6 mmol/L above their current
blood sugar trigger. Foods that raise your blood sugar a lot AND
keep them elevated for a long time (i.e., fat+carb combo foods) are
bad news.

Significantly elevated blood sugars after meals outside the healthy
range is a sign that you are overfilling your carb fuel tank AND
that your body fat stores are full. We do not recommend people
aim for flatline blood sugars as it can lead to simply swapping
carbohydrates for low satiety nutrient-poor added fats.

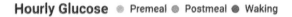

Hourly Glucose   Premeal   Postmeal   Waking

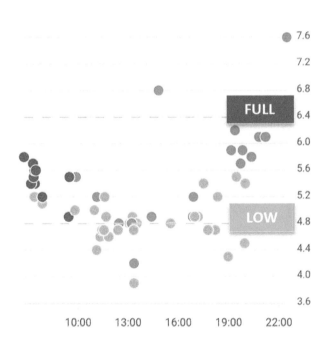

So, once your blood sugars are in the healthy range, the next step is
to simply delay or skip meals to allow your premeal blood sugar to

drop below Your Personalised Trigger. Combined with protein/nutrient focused meals, this allows both your fat and glucose stores to be depleted.

The Bottom Line

- Lower and stable blood sugar and insulin levels are a sign of good metabolic health but managing the symptoms with a high-fat diet does not lead to greater metabolic health.
- Rather than focusing on avoiding short-term blood sugar and insulin spikes, you should focus on higher satiety, nutrient-dense foods that will reduce your cravings and allow you to lose body fat.

Keto Lie #11: You Should 'Eat Fat to Satiety' to Lose Body Fat

———————— ⚜ ————————

This is perhaps one of the most seductive lies that I fell for in the early days of my low-carb/keto journey.

I kept hearing the keto gurus say that I should simply 'eat fat to satiety'. Apparently, fat was the most satiating macronutrient and the best thing I could choose to eat if I wanted to get skinny and avoid my family history of Type 2 Diabetes.

However, after putting this into practice and gaining even more fat on my body, it was time to see if this holds up against the data.

What is Satiety?

Satiety is the feeling of fullness (i.e., satisfaction) after a meal. A satiating meal will empower you to feel full with less energy (calories) and stop you from feeling hungry for longer.

Satiety is the holy grail of sustainable energy balance and fat loss.

Unless you are living in a metabolic ward with all your food provided or can track your energy in vs energy out perfectly all the time and fight against your appetite (which you can't), prioritising foods that leave you fuller with less energy is critical to ensuring you achieve the outcomes you want.

Food manufacturers have worked out how to create foods that minimise satiety and make us eat more of them. However, we can reverse engineer our food choices to choose foods that will enable us to feel full and stop eating before we consume excess calories.

In addition to macronutrients (i.e. protein, fibre, carbs and fat) and micronutrients (i.e. vitamins, minerals, amino acids and fatty acids), there are <u>other factors such as texture, smell and taste,</u> which are all somewhat interrelated.

These factors, combined with the dopamine hit these foods provide, have ensured that we seek out these foods. However, these senses can become maladaptive to our detriment in an environment where food is cheap and plentiful and engineered for greater palatability and lower satiety.

Back in 1995, a study was done at the University of Sydney that quantified the satiety response to 1000 kJ (239 calories) portions of 38 different foods (refer *A Satiety Index of Common Foods*). The outcomes of this study are shown in the chart below.

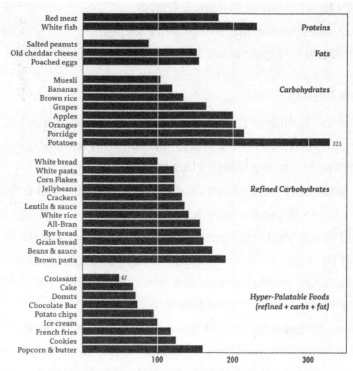

Holt, S.H., Miller, J.C., Petocz, P., Farmakalidis, E. (Department of Biochemistry, University of Sydney, Australia.) "A satiety index of common foods." European Journal of Clinical Nutrition, Volume 49, September 1995, pages 675-690.

The cooked and cooled plain potato (with lots of resistant starch) had the highest satiety response, while the croissant had the lowest satiety response. While there are only 38 data points, this laboratory data can give us a sense of how different macronutrients (or combinations) affect our satiety signals.

Does Eating More Fat Help Us Eat Less?

When we plot fat vs satiety score from the Holt (1995) study, we see that:

- very low-fat foods are harder to overeat.
- higher fat foods like egg and cheese are more satiating than those that are a combination of fat and carbs together; and
- foods that are a mix of fat and carbs (e.g., cake and doughnuts) are the least satiating.

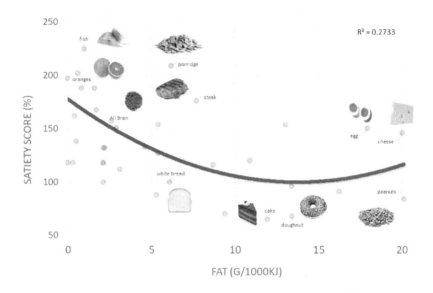

When we look at the satiety response to fat based on our analysis of half a million days of people using MyFitnessPal, as shown in this next chart, we see that lower-fat foods provide greater satiety than higher fat foods on a calorie-for-calorie basis.

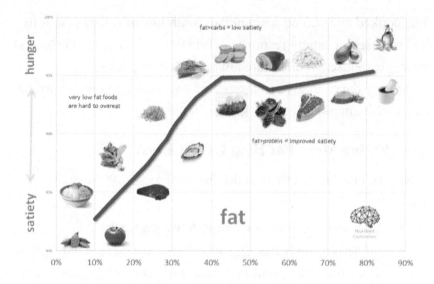

The satiety response curves from our analysis data from people using Nutrient Optimiser show a similar trend. When we consume foods with a higher percentage of fat, we consume more calories.

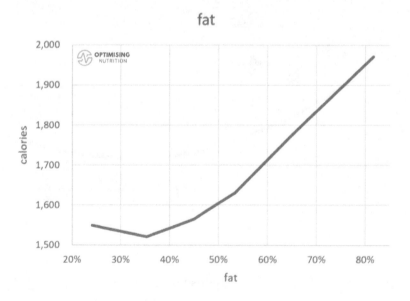

So, it seems the three separate data sets indicate that higher fat foods are not satiating. Despite the common belief that you should 'eat fat to satiety', adding more dietary fat will not lead to greater satiety or help us to lose fat from our bodies. While eating fat may cause us to burn more fat, the fat we burn will be from our food, not our body.

Higher Fat Foods are Not as Nutrient-Dense

When we look at fat vs nutrient density, we see that higher fat foods tend to contain less-essential nutrients per calorie. While fat can be a great source of energy, very high-fat foods often do not provide us with as much of the nutrients we need to thrive.

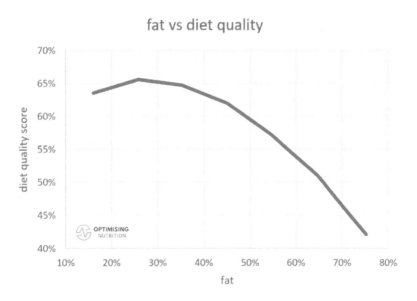

Are we getting fat from eating more fat or carbs?

The following chart shows the change in energy from each of the macronutrients in the food system over the last century. While carbs (red line) have increased over the past 50 years, the amount of fat (blue line) has been steadily on the increase over the past century.

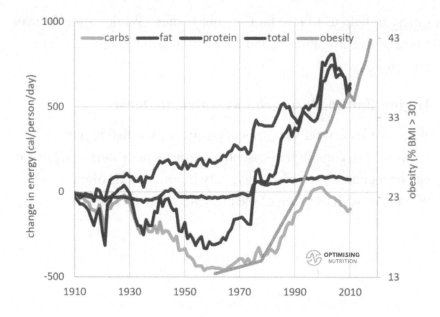

Ever since we worked out how to extract oil from soybeans, corn and rapeseed in 1908, the amount of fat in our diet has steadily risen. Combined with the large-scale farming practices and agricultural subsidies implemented in the 1960s, the availability of calories per person (mainly from fat and carbohydrates, not protein) has skyrocketed.

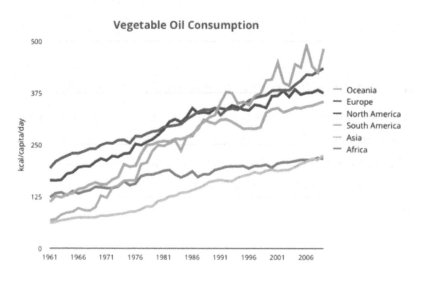

The following chart shows the change in calories and obesity rates since 1960. Protein (green line) has only increased marginally, while both fat (blue line) and carbs (red line) have increased a LOT. Overall, since the lows of the 1960s, energy availability has increased by about 1000 calories per day per person in the US, with similar trends occurring across the globe.

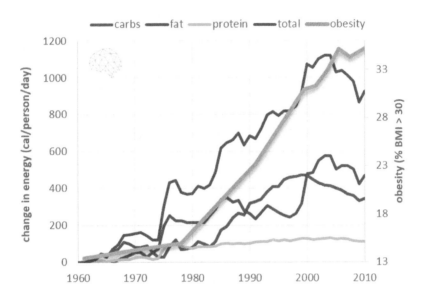

But, before we declare that all fat is bad, we need to look at where that extra fat has come from. When we look at the growth in fat consumed, we see the increase in 'salad and cooking oils' tracks closely with obesity, while animal-based added fat sources (e.g., butter, dairy and lard) have not changed significantly since 1970.

The increase in easily accessible energy from both refined grains and refined fats from large-scale agriculture is the smoking gun or the 'elephant in the room' of the obesity epidemic.

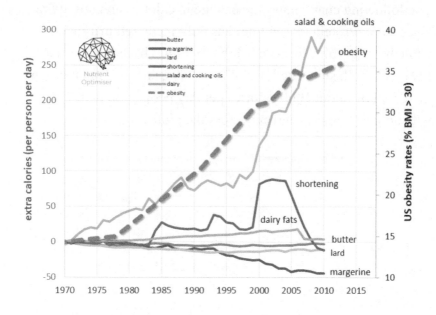

Omega-3 fatty acids

Things get more interesting when we look at the satiety response to each type of fat.

The chart below shows the satiety response to omega-3 fatty acids from 40,000 days of data from people using Nutrient Optimiser. Once we get an omega-3 intake of more than 3 g/2000 calories, we see improved satiety. Our satiety response to foods that contain more omega-3 fatty acids starts to taper off beyond around 7 g/2000 calories. So, there's not much use pushing our omega-3 intake higher than this.

The most plentiful and bioavailable source of omega-3 is fatty fish (e.g., salmon, mackerel, sardines, halibut, arctic char, lingcod and caviar). While plant-based foods contain some omega-3 as alpha-linolenic acid (ALA), humans are not good at converting it to bioactive forms (i.e., DHA and EPA). Consuming fatty fish and other seafood gives us a better chance of absorbing the omega-3 into our cells where it is required.

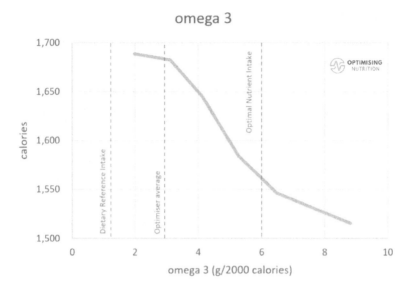

Some examples of popular omega-3 sources (along with the amount of omega 3 they contain as a percentage of energy) include:

- caviar (23%)
- sardines (7%)
- oyster (6%)
- salmon (5%)
- mussels (5%)
- tuna (2%)
- shrimp (2%)
- scallops (2%)
- cod (1%)

However, while omega-3 is essential, you're unlikely to get all of the satiety and health benefits from simply taking omega-3 supplements. Foods that are high in omega-3 provide many other beneficial micronutrients, so you should do everything you can to meet your omega-3 target from food.

Cholesterol

Cholesterol is a controversial nutrient with a chequered history. We need some dietary cholesterol to build our cell membranes and make hormones. However, in the past, it was thought that dietary cholesterol contributes to cholesterol in the blood, which was associated with heart disease.

The American Heart Association set a limit on cholesterol of 300 mg per day, and since the 1950s, the US population dutifully reduced their intake of dietary cholesterol. Unfortunately, as you can see from this chart, this reduction in dietary cholesterol has tracked in the opposite direction of the obesity epidemic.

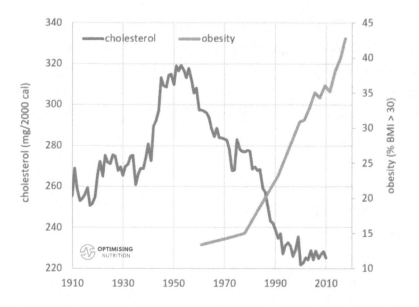

Interestingly, the 2015 Dietary Guidelines quietly removed cholesterol as a 'nutrient of concern' due to the lack of evidence that it increased the risk of heart disease as previously thought. However, it turns out that your liver regulates the cholesterol in your blood, and the levels are not strongly correlated with dietary intake.

Our satiety analysis suggests that people tend to eat less when they consume food that contains more cholesterol. It appears that your body craves cholesterol and encourages you to continue eating cholesterol-containing foods until you get enough. Ironically, the lower limit targeted by the American Heart Association and the Dietary Guidelines aligns with the lowest satiety response!

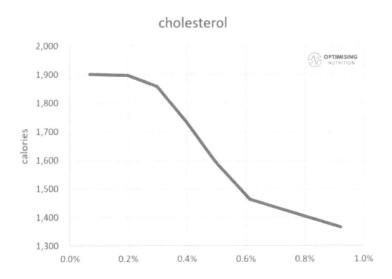

Popular foods that contain more cholesterol are listed below. These are generally nutritious foods and should not be avoided due to fear of their high cholesterol content.

- egg yolk (3.0%)
- liver (3.0%)
- whole egg (2.3%)
- caviar (2.0%)
- shrimp (1.6%)
- oyster (0.7%)
- fish oil (0.5%)
- cod (0.5%)
- pork (0.4%)
- salmon (0.4%)

As with omega-3s, it's unlikely you'll benefit as much if you try to increase your cholesterol in the absence of whole food. Food like eggs, liver and seafood contain cholesterol in a matrix of many other beneficial nutrients. There is no reason to avoid these nutritious foods simply because they contain cholesterol.

Saturated Fat

The data from the USDA Economic Research Service indicates that our intake of saturated fat has increased over the last century, but not as much as the mono and polyunsaturated fats.

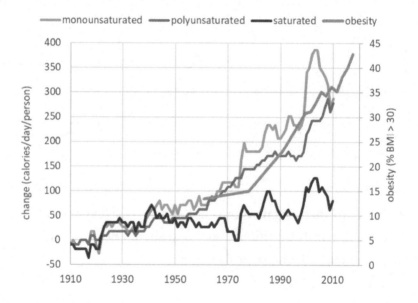

In percentage terms, saturated fat has decreased significantly since the 1930s.

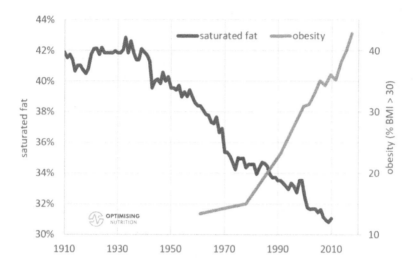

Over the past half-century, our intake of foods that contain more saturated fat (e.g., dairy, butter and lard) has not changed significantly. In contrast, our use of unsaturated 'salad and cooking oils' (i.e., oils extracted from soy, canola and corn as used as an ingredient in our food) has skyrocketed!

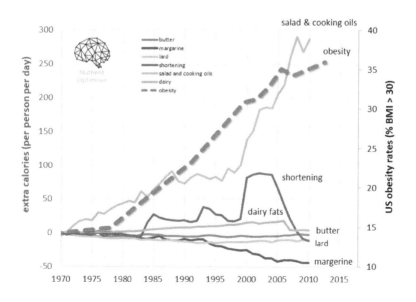

The satiety response chart shown below indicates that we eat more when we consume more saturated fat, but only up until about 30% of calories. This decrease at higher levels may be due to the fact that foods that contain more saturated fat also tend to contain more bioavailable protein.

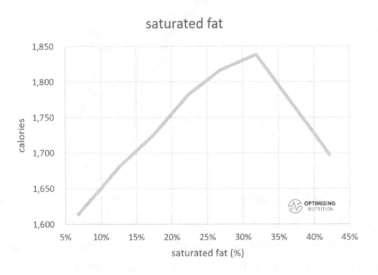

Examples of popular foods that contain more saturated fat include:
- coconut oil (83%),
- butter (57%),
- lard (47%),
- Parmesan cheese (33%),
- bacon (33%),
- ground beef (27%),
- Brazil nuts (22%), and
- eggs (20%).

While you probably don't need to prioritise more saturated fats if you are trying to lose weight, there is no need to actively avoid nutritious foods that contain saturated fat (e.g., eggs, cheese and meat).

Monounsaturated fat

Over the past century, the availability of polyunsaturated and monounsaturated fats in our food system has both increased by 300 to 400 calories per person per day, while saturated fat has increased by about 100 calories per day.

The satiety response chart below shows we tend to consume about 25% more energy when our diet contains more monounsaturated fat.

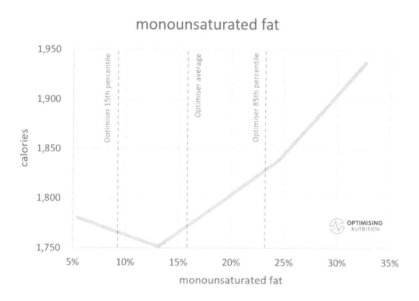

To put this into context, popular foods that contain more monounsaturated fats include:

- olive oil (74%),
- avocado oil (72%),
- avocados (55%),
- pecans (53%),
- almonds (49%),
- lard (45%),
- cashews (40%),

- peanuts (39%), and
- bacon (38%).

Although many of these are low-carb and keto favourites, they are not going to be optimal if your goal is to lose body fat. Even worse than naturally occurring fat is when seed oils are combined with starches and sugars.

Polyunsaturated Fat

Although it makes up a smaller portion of our energy intake than monounsaturated fats, our consumption of polyunsaturated fats has followed a similar trajectory over the last century.

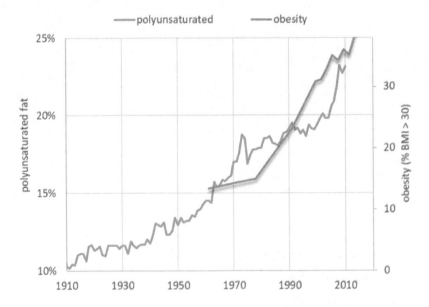

Our analysis shows that calories increase rapidly once polyunsaturated fats contribute more than 10% of calories.

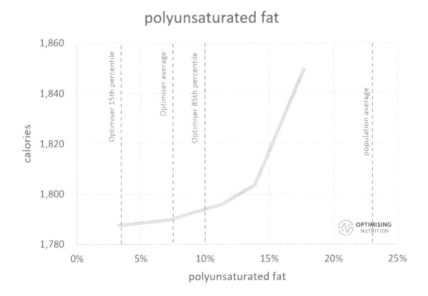

Popular foods that contain more polyunsaturated fat include:

- walnuts (65%),
- mayonnaise (59%),
- flaxseeds (48%),
- Brazil nuts (33%),
- pecans (28%), and
- peanuts (33%).

As an aside, an interesting study looked at the response to 70% fat diets with high levels of polyunsaturated fats vs saturated fats (see *Differential metabolic effects of saturated versus polyunsaturated fats in ketogenic diets*). Participants saw more elevated blood ketones, lower glucose and better insulin resistance on the diet that provided more energy from polyunsaturated fats compared to saturated fats.

According to Dr Tommy Wood, it appears that polyunsaturated fats allow us to eat more and put on more body fat before we exceed our Personal Fat Threshold and become insulin resistant. A ketogenic diet consisting of less saturated fat and more polyunsaturated fat may be helpful if your goal is simply to maximise ketone levels for therapeutic purposes. However, it may not be ideal for body composition or long-term health.

A diet with less unsaturated fat may help raise our Personal Fat Threshold, so we don't become insulin resistant and develop Type 2 Diabetes as quickly.

However, our satiety analysis indicates that unsaturated fats may also drive us to consume more energy from refined fat, which will cause us to gain fat more quickly and eventually reach our Personal Fat Threshold.

Summary

To bring all this together, the chart below shows the satiety response curves plotted on one chart.

- Foods that contain more omega-3 fatty acids and cholesterol tend to be more satiating. Avoidance of foods that are otherwise nutritious and contain energy, such as cholesterol or omega-3, may have a negative impact on satiety.
- Monounsaturated, saturated, and polyunsaturated fats all have a negative impact on satiety. However, monounsaturated fat tends to align with the greatest energy intake.

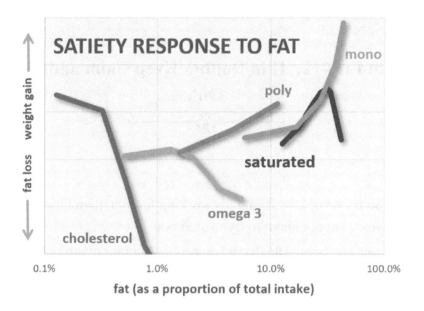

Keto Lie #12: If in Doubt, 'Keep Calm and Keto On'.

———————— ⚜ ————————

I f you try keto, love it, and it's working for you, then more power to you! I'm not about to try to stop you.

However, the typical advice when people run into roadblocks with their keto diet is to 'eat more fat to raise ketones' and 'keep calm and keto on'.

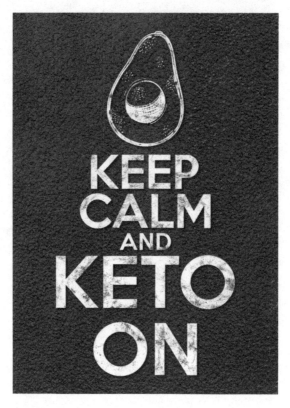

If you have plenty of ketones but are still not losing weight, it might be helpful to dig a little deeper to understand what is happening and how you can tweak your diet to ensure you start moving towards your goals.

This final chapter digs into the concept of oxidative priority to understand how your body uses available fuels and how you can intelligently manage the inputs of the various fuels based on your body's requirements to get the outputs you want.

Oxidative Priority

To understand why 'keto' fails for some people, it's helpful to understand a little more about how your body uses fuel. As mentioned in Lie #5, oxidative priority refers to the order in which you use the fuels available to your body (i.e. alcohol, ketones, glucose, protein and fat).

Imagine if you poured crude oil on the ground, poured petrol on top of it, and lit a match. The petrol would burn off quickly while the oil may not even ignite. This is because oil burns slowly, while petrol burns rapidly.

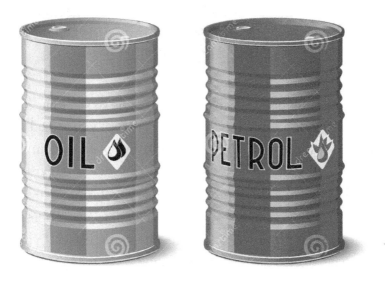

Volatile fuels like gas are hard to store. By contrast, it's easier to store large amounts of energy as unrefined crude oil. The more we refine these fuels, the easier they are to burn. Similarly, the degree of refining and the balance of macronutrients causes the fuels in your body to behave differently.

The fact that different macronutrients are harder to convert to usable energy and there are more losses in their conversion goes by several names, including:

- the thermic effect of food,
- dietary-induced thermogenesis, or
- the specific dynamic action of food.

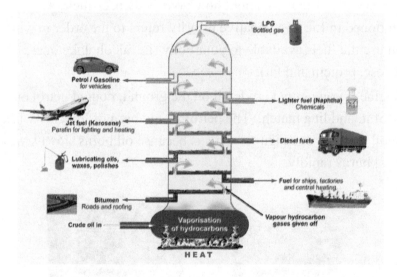

Most of us do not overeat protein because it is so satiating. Your appetite for high-protein foods shuts down once you've had enough. It is more difficult for our body to convert protein to energy (ATP), so it is a poor energy source for everyday use.

This means that our two remaining primary fuel sources are carbs and fat. Although your body needs to maintain *some* glucose in your bloodstream, you won't burn the fat in your blood if you already have excess glucose in circulation.

Because you can only store about 5 g of glucose in your blood (about a teaspoon's worth), a little dietary carbohydrate can quickly change your blood sugar levels (particularly if your liver and muscles are already full of glycogen and your fat stores are also full).

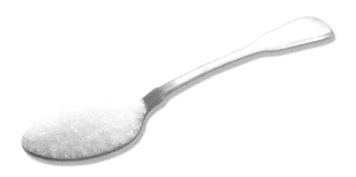

We can convert sugar to fat (via de novo lipogenesis), but most of the time, it's the fat in our diet that is stored because your body tries to burn off the glucose first, and any leftover dietary fat can easily be stored.

It's not necessarily that fat is a better fuel source than carbs, but it's the glucose that will show up in your bloodstream and register on your meter after you eat. Glucose essentially floats on top of the fat in your bloodstream and your adipose tissue.

So, to access your body fat, you need first to deplete both the glucose and fat from your blood.

In your body, your fuel tanks are separate but interconnected. As you deplete the glucose in your blood, it will be refilled from the glycogen stores in your liver (note: glycogen is just the fancy name for the storage form of glucose), and the glycogen stores in your muscles will be reduced. As the glycogen in your liver becomes depleted and you can no longer easily top up the glucose in your blood, your body will turn to the fat in your blood, and then finally, your body fat.

You can think of your available fuels as though they are stacked up on top of each other (as shown below).

glucose in the blood

â

liver glycogen

â

free fatty acids in your blood

â

body fat

So, when you measure blood glucose, you are not just measuring the sugar in your blood. You are really measuring all the fuels stacked up in your body. If your glucose is high, all the other fuel tanks are also full to the brim!

What Does This Mean for You?

- You have very little room to store alcohol or ketones. In addition, they are more volatile than other fuels, so they must be used first.
- Most of the protein you eat is used for muscle protein synthesis (MPS) and other critical bodily functions.
- While 'excess protein' not used in MPS *can* be converted to energy (ATP), this usually only happens when you are not eating enough carbs to supply your body with glucose. Your body will then use the protein in your diet to make the glucose it requires via gluconeogenesis. If you are under consuming dietary protein, it will use the protein on your body (i.e., muscles) as a last resort.

- Excess protein (i.e., that is not required for muscle repair and other bodily functions) can be excreted in the urine (i.e., it is not used for energy). A little bit of 'labile protein' circulates in your bloodstream, but not much.

- Protein has the highest thermic effect (i.e. 20 to 35% of energy is lost in the conversion to usable energy), so your body has to work hard to convert it to use for energy. We don't usually consume 'excess protein'. Your body prefers to get energy from fat and/or carbs, so higher protein foods tend to be more satiating once you've had enough.

- Your body has *some* capacity to store glucose in the liver, blood and muscle, but not a lot compared to your body fat stores.

- You have some fatty acids in your bloodstream to use for fuel but an enormous capacity to store excess energy that you do not use.

- The amount of energy your liver drip feeds into your bloodstream from day to day is tiny compared to the amount of energy you store as fat.

- Some people can hold a tremendous amount of fat in their fatty tissue before it backs up and overflows into their bloodstream (i.e., insulin resistance, pre-diabetes or Type 2 Diabetes).

- Meanwhile, due to genetics and other factors, other people have a much smaller ultimate capacity in their fat cells before it overflows (i.e., they develop Type 2 Diabetes even though on the outside they appear thin). This difference in fat storage capacity is known as the Personal Fat Threshold.

- You need to deplete the upstream fuels before your body uses that unwanted fat on your butt and your belly.

Baseline – Modern Processed Diet

To help unpack what this means in practical terms, the diagrams below show you how you can unlock each of these fuel tanks and burn your body fat. Alcohol, ketones, and protein are not generally significant fuel sources. Therefore, we only need to focus on glucose and fat.

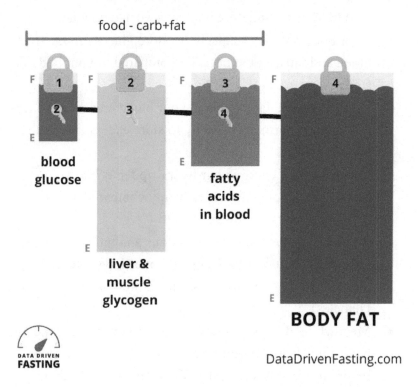

The body has four main storage compartments for energy – blood glucose, liver and muscle glycogen, fatty acids in the blood and body fat. These storage containers are all separate but interconnected to a degree.

You can think of the energy flowing downhill from left to right (based on oxidative priority). If one of the downstream storage containers is overfull and the upstream tanks become depleted, the energy *can* flow back upstream due to excess pressure in the other fuel tanks. For example:

- when the glucose in your blood becomes depleted, it can be replenished by the glycogen in your liver (via glycogenolysis),
- the glycerol backbone of fat can be converted to glucose (via glyceroneogenesis), and
- once the free fatty acids in your blood become depleted and you don't have excessive amounts coming in from dietary fat, they are topped up from your body fat stores (via lipolysis).

This diagram above shows glucose in your blood, glucose in your liver and muscles (stored as glycogen), fat in your blood (as fatty acids) and fat on your body as four separate tanks, all connected by a 'pipe'. You'll notice that the pipe connecting each of the fuel tanks flows downstream towards the right. You should also note that the 'pipe' is not drawn at the bottom of each tank, indicating that you don't need to empty each tank for the downstream fuels to be used but rather deplete to normal healthy levels.

When we eat nutrient-poor, hyper-palatable foods, we continually fill our fat and glucose stores at the same time, all of these fuel tanks are full, and the 'upstream' fuel sources become 'backed up', so you never need to call on your body fat for energy.

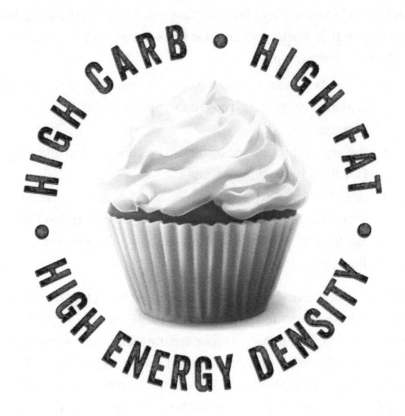

Even worse, it is so easy to overeat these highly processed, hyper-palatable foods. We have no off switch for them when they are available, so all storage tanks get full to overflowing. This leads to energy toxicity, metabolic syndrome, Type 2 Diabetes and obesity, etc.

In the following scenarios, we'll consider what happens to each of these fuel tanks when consuming one of three different dietary scenarios:

1. low-carb/high-fat.
2. low-fat/high-carb; and
3. adequate protein/lower carb/lower fat.

Scenario 1 – Low-Carb/High-Fat Diet

The good news is that when we reduce carbohydrates using a low-carb or keto diet, we can start to drain our glucose stores.

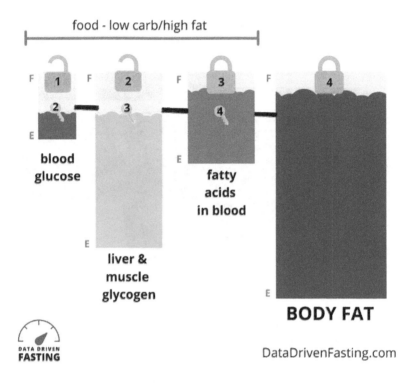

Even if you are not eating carbs, your body can always refill your blood sugar from the glycogen stores in your liver and muscles. This is why your blood sugars may continue to rise when you haven't eaten anything for quite a while.

Also, if the downstream fuel tanks are backed up with the fuel, you will still see high blood sugars. The blood sugar, glycogen and fatty acids in your blood will never go to zero because they will be topped up from the downstream storage tanks (via gluconeogenesis). This is why people with more body fat tend to have higher waking blood sugars.

Because your blood glucose is a small fuel tank (5 g of glucose or about 20 calories worth), it fills and empties quickly both before and after meals. It's also straightforward to measure using a glucose meter (also known as a glucometer) to get a precise understanding of your current energy status. When we measure glucose, we are getting a good understanding of whether all the downstream fuel tanks are also overfilled.

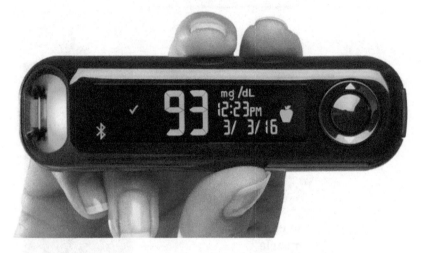

So, if your blood sugars are higher than normal for you, you are likely in an energy surplus, with plenty of fuel on board. But when your blood sugars start to drop below your normal, it may be time to eat.

Most of the time, waiting until blood glucose has fallen below their typical pre-meal blood sugar stops people from overfilling their upstream fuel tanks. This, in turn, causes your body to call on the liver and muscle glycogen to refill the blood glucose and usually forces people to deplete their fatty acids in their blood, which can be refilled from their body fat, and voila, fat loss from the body!

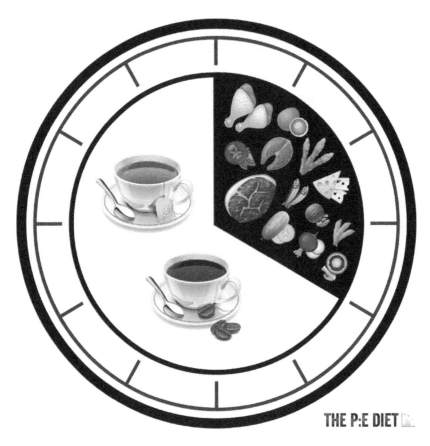

THE P:E DIET

However, some people get into trouble when they refeed with a very high-fat, low protein diet. These foods have low <u>satiety</u>, so we end up eating more of them. Therefore, we consume more calories when our diet has a higher percentage of energy from fat.

If the fat in your bloodstream is continually topped up from your diet, there is never an opportunity for body fat to flow back into the bloodstream to be used.

We have seen this in a number of people using <u>Data-Driven Fasting</u> who have very low blood sugars but are still carrying a lot of body fat. Due to a mistaken belief that fat is a 'free fuel' because it doesn't raise insulin over the short term, they are continually refilling their fat tank even though their blood sugars may look great.

When people get stuck at this point, we recommend focusing on incrementally increasing the percentage of protein in their diet by dietary fat.

This improves <u>satiety</u> and allows both the glucose and fat fuel tanks to be drained. We'll discuss this more in *Scenario 3 – Adequate Protein/Lower-Carb/Lower-Fat*, but first, let's touch on the Low-Fat/High-Carb scenario.

Scenario 2 - Low-Fat/High-Carb

In Scenario 2 (Low-Fat/High-Carb), even though blood glucose and glycogen stores are continually being filled, so long as there is only a small amount of dietary fat, blood fats will still be depleted. Hence, stored body fat will flow back into the bloodstream to be used for fuel.

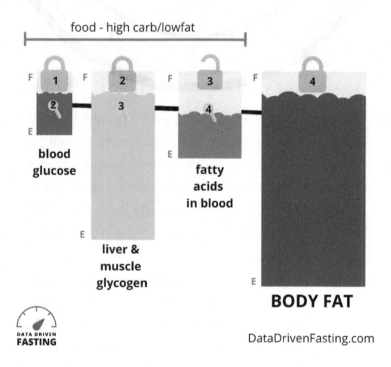

While a very low-fat diet can be useful for weight loss, the reality is that very few people (unless they adhere to an ultra-strict whole food plant-based diet) can sustain a diet with low enough levels of fat to drive fat loss over the long term.   Unfortunately, they tend to gravitate back to foods that are a mixture of carbs and fat, which allows us to consume more calories as we fill all fuel tanks at the same time.

The majority of our modern processed, packaged foods are a combination of starch, sugar and fat from vegetable oil that makes refined fat hard to escape for most people.

Scenario 3 – Adequate Protein/Lower Carb/Lower Fat

In this scenario, we have a diet that is lower in fat and lower in carbohydrates with adequate protein. This style of diet tends to have a higher nutrient density than the other scenarios. We are satiated when we have met our nutritional requirements. Once we have obtained the nutrients we need, we are less likely to continue eating.

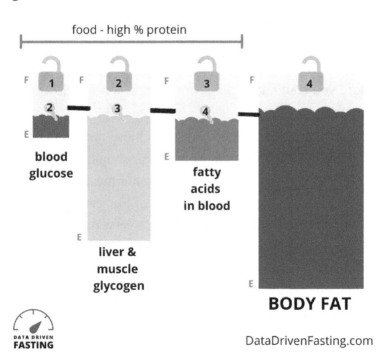

When we eat, we need to get sufficient protein and nutrients. You can think of carbs and fat as fuel, and we don't need as much of it if we are already carrying a lot of unwanted body fat on our body and a build-up of glucose in our liver and blood.

As we dial back both dietary fat and dietary carbs, we deplete the carb and fat fuel tanks in our body, and our body fat can flow back into the bloodstream to be used.

Foods with a higher protein percentage and higher nutrient density tend to be very hard to overeat. So, in time, the body fat has an opportunity to flow back into our bloodstream from storage.

While you don't have to jump to a super high-protein extreme, slowly dialling back your easily accessible energy from both carbs and fat (while still getting adequate protein and nutrients) is THE SECRET to ensuring fat loss from your body.

If we can progressively increase the percentage of protein in the diet (by reducing energy from both carbs and fat), we will tend to consume fewer calories as we drain our carb and fat fuel tanks.

How to Ensure You Continue to Make Progress

To ensure you continue to make progress, you can follow the following steps.

1. First, dial back refined carbs to achieve non-diabetic blood sugar variability. Your blood sugar should not rise more than 1.6 mmol/L or 30 mg/dL or after meals most of the time. This is where the "magic" of low-carb and keto happens. This doesn't have to be a very low-carb, high-fat or keto diet, just enough to stabilise blood sugars and reduce cravings that occur when blood sugars plummet below normal.

2. Next, we can use meal timing and the elimination of snacks to continue the fat loss journey. You can use your blood sugar as a fuel gauge to validate your hunger. In our Data

Driven Fasting Challenges, we tend to see active people consume two or three meals a day with less active people opting for one or two meals per day guided by their blood sugars.

3. If you are not achieving weight loss or your waking blood sugar is not decreasing with a main meal and a discretionary meal, it's likely that you are consuming excessive amounts of dietary fat. You should look to increase your protein percentage, food quality and nutrient density by reducing the foods that provide more energy from fat in your diet. We focus on this more in our Macros Masterclass and Micros Masterclass.

This approach is summarised in the table below.

Step	Limit	Description	When to progress
1. Stabilise blood sugars	< 1.6 mmol/L or 30 mg/dL rise after meals	Reduce processed carbs to achieve healthy blood sugar stability.	When BG rise after meals is < 1.6 mmol/L or 30 mg/dL
2. Meal timing/intermittent fasting	One main meal with one discretionary meal (OMAD+)	Reduce the number of times you eat per day. Continue until you have one main meal with a discretionary meal that you eat based on	When average meals per day are less than 1.5.

Step	Limit	Description	When to progress
		blood sugar/weight target.	
3. Increase protein % by dialling back dietary fat.	Work up to 40-50% protein.	Slowly increase protein % (by reducing dietary fat) until weight loss re-commences.	When you have reached your target weight, body fat, waist:height or waking glucose.

Resources

If you've made it this far through Big Fat Keto Lies, hopefully, you can see that:

- there are a number of moving parts to <u>Nutritional Optimisation</u> that can appear complex, and
- your nutritional prescription needs to be personalised to your current situation, goals and diet.

To help people implement the theory, we've been developing several tools that we're excited to share to help you on your journey.

Join our Community!

If you want to dive a little deeper into our world, we'd love you to join our free <u>Optimising Nutrition Community here</u>. After growing a fantastic community on Facebook over the past couple of years, we decided it was time to set up our own space away from the noise of social media.

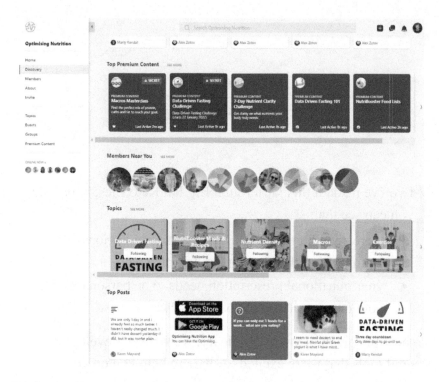

We're loving our new home away from the noise, controversies and distraction of social media. All our future challenges will be run here. You will also get a stream of recipes and other inspiration to help you continue your journey towards optimising your nutrition in the community.

Follow Optimising Nutrition

To immerse yourself in the experience and keep up with the latest information, you can also follow us on:

- Facebook,
- Twitter,
- Instagram,
- YouTube, and
- Pinterest.

We also have the following Facebook Groups:

- Optimising Nutrition Facebook Group,
- Data-Driven Fasting Facebook Group,
- Nutrient Optimiser Facebook Group, and
- NutriBooster Recipes.

Data-Driven Fasting

Measuring your blood sugar gives you an instantaneous measure of your current energy status (i.e., full or empty and needing to refuel). It enables you to solve the energy balance equation without tracking everything you eat.

We've been stunned by how well people have taken to Data-Driven Fasting. It seems most people would prefer to test their blood sugars a couple of times a day than trying to solve the calories in vs calories out equation.

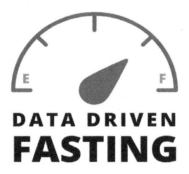

Data-Driven Fasting is a great way to get started in your journey towards optimising your blood sugars, weight and health.

If you want to identify your *personalised trigger*, you can download the free baselining spreadsheet here or the 190-page manual here to learn all about Data-Driven Fasting.

To continue, you can choose the 30 Day Challenge or the self-guided Program.

Check your macros

If you find your blood sugars are great, but your fat loss has stalled, many people find it helpful to check their current macro intake. You can use our free macro calculator to find your target macros.

Progressively dialling up protein percentage (by decreasing fat and/or carbs) tends to work wonders for most people and enables them to regain control of their appetite.

7 Day-Nutrient Clarity Challenge

If you want to fine-tune your nutrient density by adding in foods and meals that contain more of the nutrients you aren't getting enough of, you can take our Free 7 Day Food Discovery Challenge here.

NutriBooster Recipe Books

After publishing hundreds of articles about nutrient density, satiety, and optimising blood sugar and insulin levels, we finally realised that if nutritional optimisation was going to become a movement, we needed to make it as easy as possible for YOU to implement in your kitchen.

NutriBooster Recipes

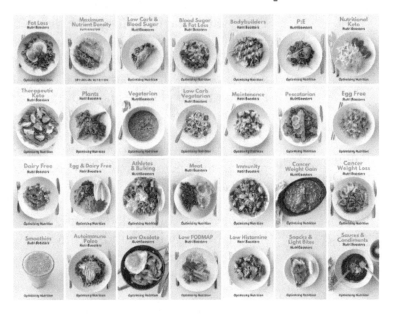

When everything these days is optimised using artificial intelligence and big data, why shouldn't you be able to optimise the nutrients in your food? Our ambitious goal was to reinvent and revolutionise the recipe genre by bringing the essential micronutrients into the spotlight using a data-driven approach. So, we created a series of recipe books tailored to a range of goals.

To help you decide, we have prepared this table with a brief description of each book and who it would be appropriate for.

Goal	Appropriate for
Fat Loss	Designed for rapid fat loss, with plenty of protein for satiety and to prevent muscle loss, micronutrients to minimise cravings and less energy from carbs and dietary fat to lower blood glucose and allow you to use your body fat for fuel.
Maximum Nutrient Density	These are the most nutrient-dense recipes to pack all the micronutrients you need into your calorie budget.
Low Carb & Blood Sugar	Designed to stabilise blood sugars and maintain weight on a nutritious low-carb diet. Ideal for someone with diabetes or anyone who enjoys eating low-carb.
Blood Sugar & Fat Loss	Designed for someone with elevated blood sugars and body fat to lose.
Bodybuilders	Designed for someone looking to gain muscle without increasing excess body fat. They provide plenty of micronutrients, with enough energy to support your workouts, but not so much you'll end up with a 'dirty bulk'.
High Protein:Energy	Designed with a high protein:energy ratio for aggressive fat loss. These are ideal for an aggressive short term PSMF style diet for rapid fat loss.
Nutritional Keto	Designed for someone who enjoys keto but does *not* require therapeutic ketone levels.
Therapeutic Keto	Designed for people who require therapeutic ketone levels for specific

Goal	Appropriate for
	conditions (e.g., for epilepsy, dementia, or Parkinson's).
Plant-Based	The most nutrient-dense plant-based recipes available.
Vegetarian	The most nutrient-dense vegetarian meals.
Low Carb Vegetarian	These are the most nutrient-dense, low-carb vegetarian meals designed to stabilise blood sugars.
Lacto Vegetarian	These are the most nutrient-dense, lacto vegetarian (i.e., no meat, seafood or eggs).
Maintenance	Designed to help you maintain your body weight by optimising nutrient content to live a healthy and energised life.
Pescatarian	These are the most nutrient-dense pescatarian recipes (i.e., vegetarian plus seafood).
Egg-Free	The most nutrient-dense meals without eggs.
Dairy-Free	The most nutrient-dense meals without dairy.
Egg & Dairy-Free	The most nutrient-dense meals without eggs or dairy.
Athletes & Bulking	Recipes design to provide enough energy to support your activity, growth and recovery while still providing plenty of essential nutrients.

Goal	Appropriate for
Meat-Based	These are the most nutrient-dense meals that contain meat (i.e., beef, pork, chicken, etc.).
Immunity	Recipes designed to prioritise nutrients like iron, selenium, zinc, potassium, vitamin A, C, and D that support healthy immune function.
Cancer (Weight Loss & Nutrient Density)	Designed for someone with cancer by providing less glutamic acid and methionine while maximising nutrient density and satiety to promote fat loss.
Cancer (Weight Maintenance)	Designed for someone with cancer that requires less glutamic acid and methionine while providing enough energy to maintain a healthy weight.
Cancer (Weight Gain)	Designed for someone with cancer that requires less glutamic acid and methionine while providing plenty of energy to support weight gain after or during cancer treatment.
Smoothies	The most nutritious smoothies for quick and easy meals on the go.
Low Oxalate	Low-oxalate NutriBoosters to maximise nutrient density while minimising oxalates.
Low FODMAP	Designed to maximise nutrient density and satiety while avoiding high FODMAP foods.
Low Histamine	Designed to histamines while maximising nutrient density as much as possible.

Goal	Appropriate for
Low Fat	Ideal for people who prefer a low-fat diet or need to quickly refill glycogen stores when your blood sugars are low or after a workout.

Each book contains 33 recipes plus an index of links to 100+ additional secret recipes that align with your chosen goal. When you purchase one of the books, you will receive:

- an e-book with **the most nutritious meals** optimised for your goal (that you can take with you anywhere on your phone or tablet),
- a secret index of links to the **100+ most nutrient-dense recipes** optimised for your goal on our website so you will never run out of nutritious ideas to try,
- a **full micronutrient breakdown** showing the vitamins, minerals, essential fatty acids and amino acids that you will obtain from each recipe,
- access to all recipes **pre-logged in Cronometer** for your convenience, and
- a list of the **most popular nutrient-dense foods** that align with your goal.

Macros Masterclass

There is no perfect one-size-fits-all dietary prescription that works for everyone all the time. We all require a unique mix of protein, fat, and carbs tailored to our unique lifestyle, goals, budget, beliefs, and preferences.

Sadly, we've seen so much confusion and frustration as people try to follow the latest popular extreme approach, whether that be:

- Low-fat,
- Low-carb,

- Keto,
- Low protein,
- High protein,
- Plant-based, or
- Carnivore.

Even if they help for a while, the reality is that very few people manage to stick to these ways of eating long term. Instead, we usually revert to our old habits.

You don't have to upend everything you're already doing. You only need to make just enough change to start moving towards your goal at a sustainable rate.

While many people think they want overnight success. But overnight success rarely lasts. Instead, it's the incremental changes that lead to tiny habits that, before you know it, will lead to your long term goal! Rather than jumping to unsustainable extremes, we always see the best results when Optimisers progressively move towards optimal.

That's why we designed the <u>Macros Masterclass</u>. We want to guide you through to dial your macronutrients to align with your unique goals, such as:

- Fat loss while maximising satiety and minimising muscle loss.
- Muscle growth while minimising fat gain.
- Healthy maintenance and aging while preventing sarcopenia and loss of lean mass.
- Blood sugar stabilisation in someone with insulin resistance, pre-diabetes, Type-2, or Type-1 diabetes.

MACROS MASTERCLASS
30-DAY CHALLENGE

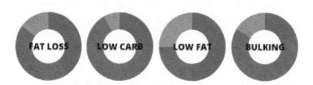

FIND THE PERFECT MIX OF PROTEIN, FAT AND CARBS TO REACH YOUR GOAL.

Our Macros Masterclass includes:

- A 30-day guided course to progressively dial in your macronutrients.
- 45 days of access to our web-based software and app, Nutrient Optimiser, which contains:
- Smart Macros Algorithm to fine-tune your macros.
- 600+ nutrient-packed NutriBooster recipes tailored for a wide range of goals and preferences.
- Optimised food lists tailored to your current diet.
- Biometric tracking.
- Training on the nuances of tracking your food to ensure you get the most out of your data.
- Access to our 600+ Nutribooster recipes in Cronometer to simplify planning ahead and tracking.
- Sample meal plans optimised for a range of goals and preferences.
- Walkthrough tutorial videos.
- Live weekly group Q&As.
- Daily posts and group support in our brand new learning platform.

The Macros Masterclass will teach you:

- The critical role of each macronutrient (protein, carbs, and fat).
- How to tailor your macros to align with your personal goals.
- To plan ahead using our NutriBooster recipes and meal plans.

In the Macros Masterclass, we will guide you through the following steps:

- Week 1 – Baselining
- Week 2 – Prioritise protein
- Week 3 – Find your carb tolerance
- Week 4 – Leverage fat

You can learn more about our Macros Masterclass, including all the FAQs here.

Micros Masterclass

We've spent the past five years researching and analysing data from people living in the real world to understand how each macronutrient and micronutrient affects their hunger and satiety.

We now have a unique database of 125,761 days of macronutrient and micronutrient data from 34,519 people who have used Nutrient Optimiser to fine-tune their diet. This has given us a unique, powerful, and precise understanding of how each micronutrient influences our cravings and how much we eat.

The key finding from our analysis is simply that humans, along with all other organisms, continually seek the nutrients they need. We continue to eat until we obtain all the nutrients we need to thrive.

In the past, it was easy to get enough nutrients, but energy (from carbs and fat) was harder to find. But today, our modern food environment is filled with calorie-dense, hyper-palatable, nutrient-poor foods that lead most of us to consume more energy than we need in our quest to obtain the nutrients we require to thrive.

Trying to deprive your body of energy is futile if you are not getting the nutrients you require daily from your food. No matter how much conscious willpower you can muster, your appetite will always win in the end!

Nutrient density is the missing piece that will empower you to gain control of your appetite. Eating a 'nutrient-dense diet' simply means getting enough of all the micronutrients you require without consuming excess energy.

We believe Nutritional Optimisation is the next big thing that many are talking about, but very few people know how to do it. That's why we created the Macros Masterclass.

MICROS MASTERCLASS
30-DAY CHALLENGE

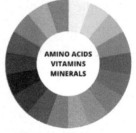

OPTIMISE YOUR DIET AT THE MICRONUTIRENT LEVEL!

Rather than depriving your body, our goal is to gamify the process of Nutritional Optimisation. Your goal is simply to solve the puzzle to give your body everything it needs to reach its full potential.

In the Micros Masterclass, we will guide you to understand which nutrients your current diet is missing and which foods and meals you can use to fill those gaps. At the end of the four weeks, you will have your own personalised shortlist list of foods and meals that you love that aligns with your goals and provide you with the nutrients your body requires to thrive.

The Micro Masterclass includes:

- A 30-day course that guides you through progressively dialling in your micronutrients.
- 45 days of access to our web-based software and app, Nutrient Optimiser, which contains:
- The Smart Macros Algorithm to fine-tune your macros.
- 600 nutrient-packed NutriBooster recipes tailored towards a wide range of goals and preferences.
- Optimised food lists tailored to your current diet.
- Biometric tracking.
- Guidance through the nuances of tracking your food to ensure you get the most out of your data.
- Access to the 600 Nutribooster recipes in Cronometer to simplify planning ahead and tracking.
- Sample meal plans optimised for varying goals and preferences.
- Weekly live group Q&As.
- Daily posts and group support in our brand-new learning platform.

The Micros Masterclass will teach you:

- The critical role each micronutrient (vitamins, minerals, amino acids, and fatty acids) plays in your diet.
- How to find all the micronutrients in the foods you eat.
- To use our NutriBooster recipes and meal plans to plan ahead.

In the Micros Masterclass, we will guide you through the following steps:

- Week 1 – Baselining to identify which nutrients your diet is lacking
- Week 2 – Optimising your minerals
- Week 3 – Optimising your Vitamins
- Week 4 – Striving for the Optimal Nutrient Intakes

You can learn more about our Micros Masterclass, including all the FAQs here.

Copyright

Legal Disclaimer and Terms of Use

This Legal Disclaimer and Terms of Use Agreement is entered into between Optimizing Nutrition and you.

All of the information provided in and throughout this book (hereafter known as Publication) and offered at https://optimisingnutrition.com/ is intended solely for general information and should NOT be relied upon for any particular diagnosis, treatment, or care.

This is not a substitute for medical advice or treatment. This Publication is only for general informational purposes. It is strongly encouraged that individuals and their families consult with qualified medical professionals for treatment and related advice on individual cases before beginning any diet.

Decisions relating to the prevention, detection, and treatment of all health issues should be made only after discussing the risks and benefits with your healthcare provider, taking into account your personal medical history, your current situation, and your future health risks and concerns.

If you are pregnant, nursing, diabetic, on medication, have a medical condition or are beginning a health or weight-control program, consult your physician before using products or services discussed in this book and before making any other dietary changes. The authors and publisher cannot guarantee the information in this Publication is safe and proper for every reader. For this reason, this Publication is sold without warranties or guarantees of any kind, express or implied, and the authors and publisher disclaim any liability, loss, or damage caused by the contents, either directly or consequentially.

Neither the US Food and Drug Administration nor any other

government regulatory body has evaluated statements made in this Publication. Products, services, and methods discussed in this publication are not intended to diagnose, treat, cure, or prevent any disease.

Indemnification

All users of this book agree to defend, indemnify, and hold harmless OptimisingNutrition.com, its contributors, any entity jointly created by them, their respective affiliates and their respective directors, officers, employees, and agents from and against all claims and expenses, including attorneys' fees, arising out of the use of this Publication.

Disclaimer of Liability

Optimizing Nutrition nor its contributors shall be held liable for any use of the information described and/or contained herein and assumes no responsibility for anyone's use of the information.

In no event shall the Optimizing Nutrition website or its contributors be liable for any direct, indirect, incidental, special, exemplary, or consequential damages (including but not limited to: procurement of substitute goods or services; loss of use, data, or profits; or business interruption) however caused and on any theory of liability, whether in contract, strict liability, tort (including negligence or otherwise), or any other theory arising in any way out of the use of this material, even if Optimizing Nutrition has been advised of the possibility of such damage.

This disclaimer of liability applies to any damages or injury, whether based on alleged breach of contract, tortious behaviour, negligence, or any other cause of action, including but not limited to damages or injuries caused by any failure of performance, error, omission, interruption, deletion, defect, delay in operation or transmission, computer virus, communication line failure, and/or theft, destruction, or unauthorized access to, alteration of, or use of any record.

Rules of Conduct: No Warranties

All content in this Publication is provided to you on an "as is," "as available" basis without warranty of any kind, either express or implied, including but not limited to the implied warranties of merchantability, fitness for a particular purpose and non-infringement.

Optimizing Nutrition makes no warranty as to the accuracy, completeness, currency, or reliability of any content available through this website. Optimizing Nutrition makes no representations or warranties of any kind that use of the website will be uninterrupted or error-free.

The user is responsible for taking all precautions necessary to ensure that any web-based content offered from the website or Publication is free of viruses.

Limitation of Liability

Optimizing Nutrition specifically disclaims any and all liability, whether based in contract, tort, strict liability or otherwise, for any direct, indirect, incidental, consequential, or special damages arising out of or in any way connected with access to or use of the website or Publication even if Optimizing Nutrition has been advised of the possibility of such damages. This limitation of liability includes, but is not limited to, reliance by any party on any content obtained through the use of this website or that arises in connection with mistakes or omissions in, or delays in transmission of information to or from the user, interruptions in telecommunications connections to this website, this Publication, or viruses, whether caused in whole or in part by negligence, acts of God, telecommunications failure, theft or destruction of or unauthorized access to the website, Publication, or related information.

Modifications

Optimizing Nutrition reserves the right to modify this Publication and the rules and regulations governing its use at any time. Modifications will be posted on the website, and users are deemed to be apprised of and bound by any changes to the website.

Your continued use of this Publication following the posting of changes to these Terms of Use constitutes your acceptance of those changes. Optimizing Nutrition may make changes in the products and/or services described in this Publication at any time.

Severability

If a section of this disclaimer is determined by any court or other competent authority to be unlawful and/or unenforceable, the other sections of this disclaimer shall continue in effect.

Thanks

Massive thanks to the following people who have played a vital role in the creation of this book.

- My wife Monica for being my muse, inspiration, supporter and partner in this journey towards Nutritional Optimisation. She has been incredibly patient and supportive as I have obsessively pursued my little hobby and used her as a guinea pig for all my latest ideas.

- Alex Zotov for saying, 'Hey, you should write a book' one Saturday morning, not to mention the constant banter and sharing of ideas to automate Nutritional Optimisation for the masses in the form of Nutrient Optimiser.

- Dr Ted Naiman for being a shining example, friend, supporter and sharing my work with his audience, not to mention letting me use all his amazing memes!

- Mike Julian, RD Dikeman, Robb Wolf, Luis Villasenor, Tyler Cartwright, Alex Leaf (aka the Insane Protein Posse) for teaching me so much through an ongoing friendship and melting pot of ideas.

- Alexandra Bucko, Dr Judi Walters, Sue Davies, Dr Jeff Gerber, Linda Fishbeck, Ellen Davis, Evdoxia Renta, Jamie Hayes, Dr Clark Connery, Alys Henderson, Melanie Avalon, Jazmine Kendall, Dr Adel Hite, Kevin Hall, Frank Plateau and Bob Farrell for their review comments in the development of this book.

- The participants in the <u>Data-Driven Fasting Challenge</u> and <u>Nutritional Optimisation Masterclass</u> who have shared their journey and their data and brought the theory to life. They have been a massive inspiration and kept me passionate and focused on my journey of learning and working to make nutritional optimisation more accessible.

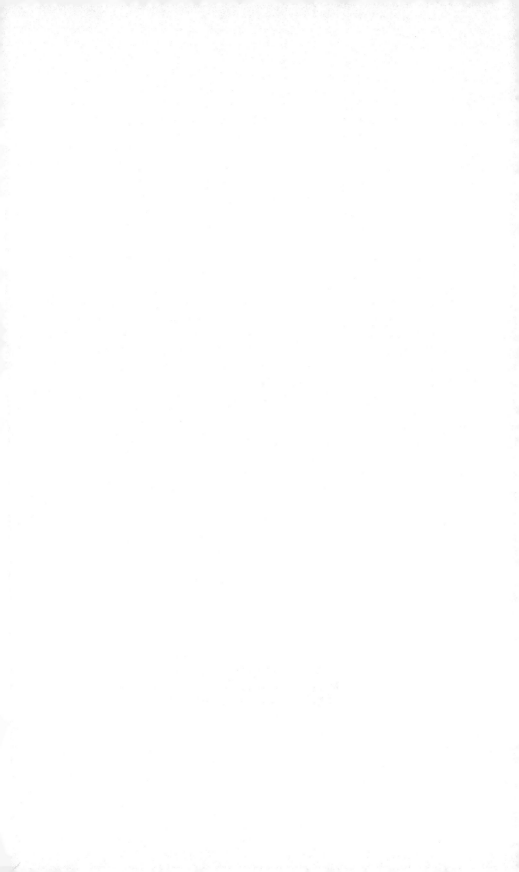

Made in the USA
Las Vegas, NV
19 November 2023

81199682R00184